It's Time to Celebrate!

We Just Turned 25,000

Just this past week, the TBI HOPE Facebook community
passed 25,000 members, making our social family
one of the world's largest online communities for those
affected by brain injury.

To those who have made our online family what
it is, a heartfelt thank you!

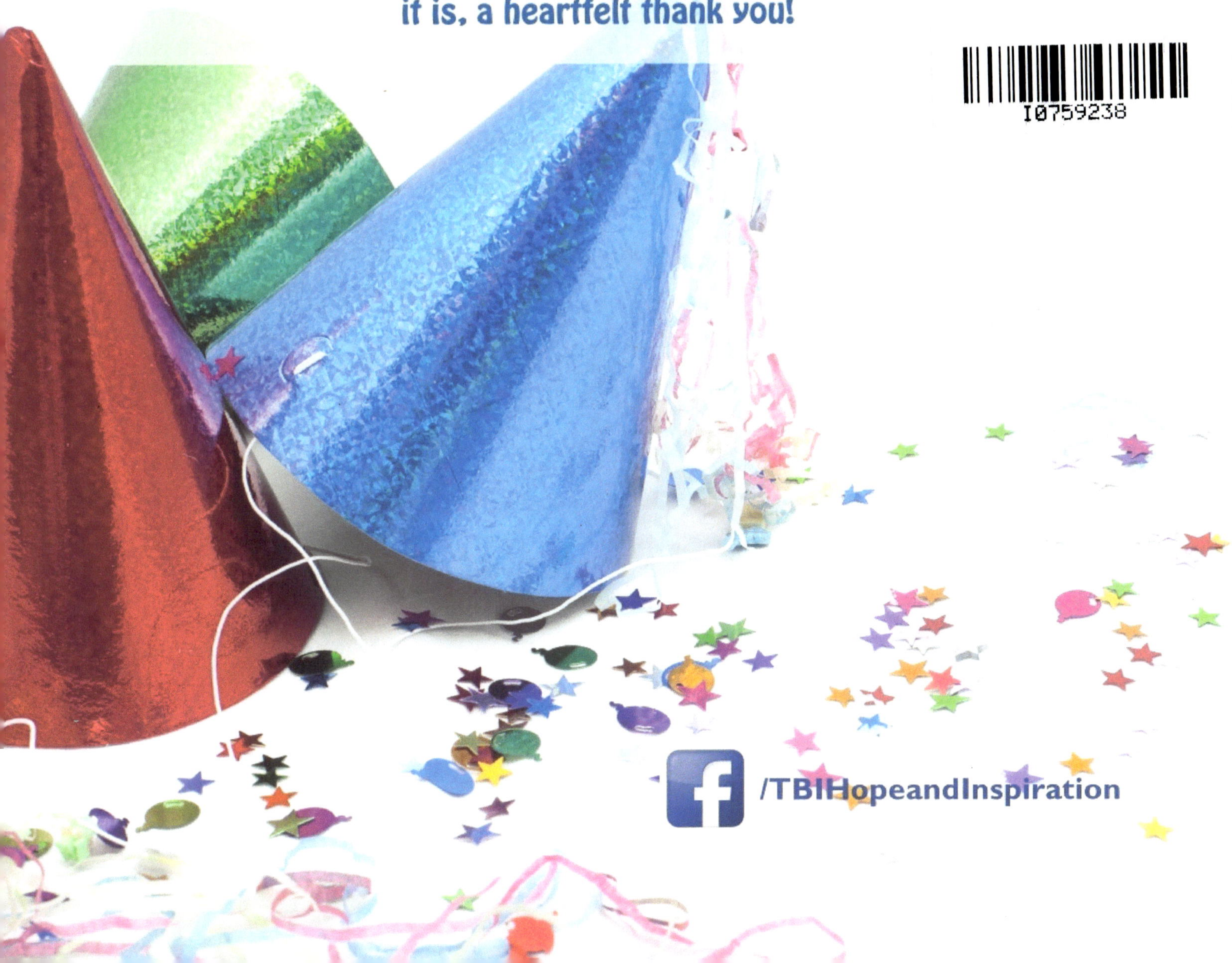

Welcome

TBI HOPE MAGAZINE

Serving All Impacted by Brain Injury

August 2017

Publisher
David A. Grant

Editor
Sarah Grant

Contributing Writers
Laura Chagnon
Nancy Hueber
Ric Johnson
Kim Maronay
Rosemary Rawlins
Jeff Sebell
Rodney Smith
Jennifer White
Karee White

Amazing Cartoonist
Patrick Brigham

FREE subscriptions at
www.TBIHopeMagazine.com

Welcome to the August 2017 issue of TBI HOPE Magazine!

We have a very exciting issue this month as we invite you to read our first-ever Editor's Choice issue. In addition to some first-time contributors, you'll have the opportunity to read a few stories from the first year of our publication. Never before in print, these are the best-of-the-best from the early years of TBI HOPE Magazine.

Also in this month's issue is a special section titled, *Is the VA Raising the Bar for Healthcare?* Traumatic Brain Injury has long been called the signature injury of today's active military, making this a timely piece.

Just a few days ago, the TBI HOPE Facebook family passed the 25,000 member mark. When I founded this online community back in early 2013, I never envisioned a community that would circle the globe with members from over forty countries worldwide. To all who have contributed to our social family in any way, a heartfelt thank you. Your experience has value and has helped others.

We hope you enjoy this issue. I welcome your feedback and suggestions as we are always trying to improve what we do. You can email me personally at david@tbihopeandinspiration.com.

Peace,

David A. Grant
Publisher

Contents

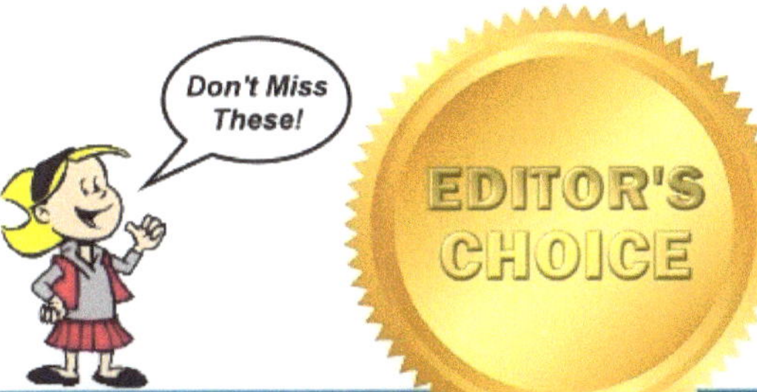

*Yesterday is not ours to recover,
but tomorrow is ours to win or lose.*
~Lyndon B. Johnson

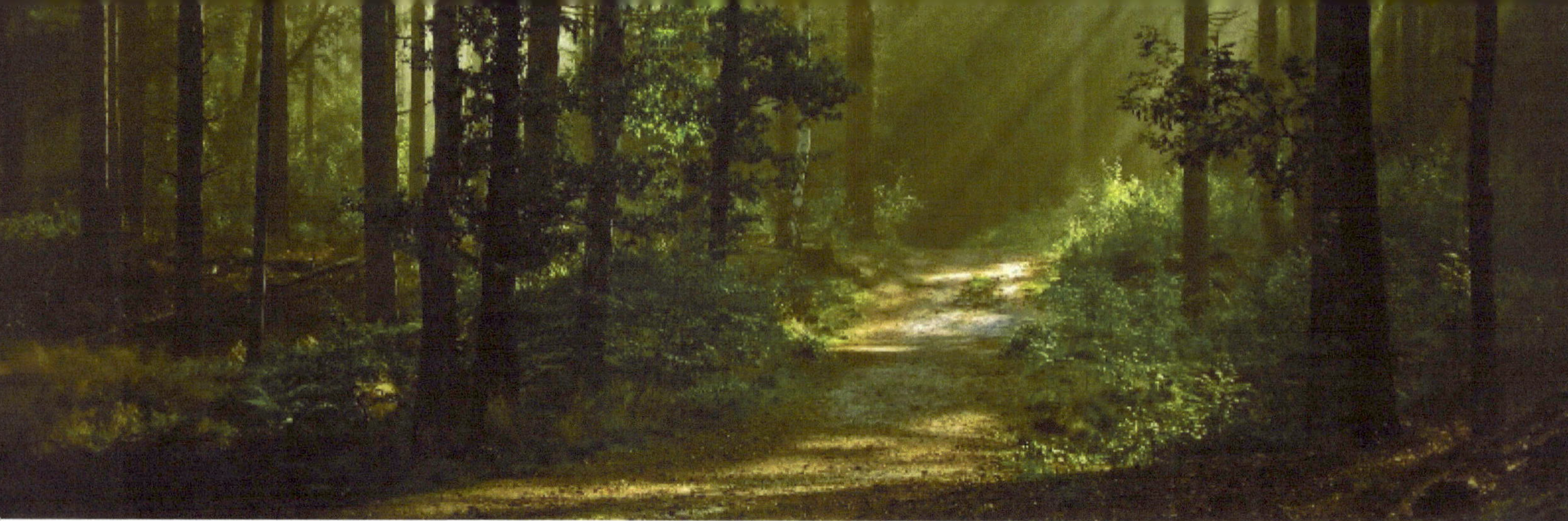

The Road Not Taken

By Ric Johnson

Robert Frost once wrote, "Take the road not taken." Well, thanks, Mr. Frost, but what road were you writing about? I'm sure it wasn't the road that all TBI survivors tread. The road we are walking on is not written on any map. It's not paved, or marked with footsteps. It's the road of our new lives.

My injury happened over thirteen years ago and it seems that instead of traveling a road, I'm breaking a new path daily. Many times I'm following steps I walked on before my injury: making breakfast; getting dressed; going to the same stores; talking to the same people, etc. Following the same old routines. But even those same old chores can really be brand new as we have to figure out exactly what that chore entails.

Let's talk about yesterday's coffee. 1) Find the coffee and filter – check. 2) Place filter and coffee into the coffee maker – check. 3) Fill the pot with cold water – check. 4) Empty water into the coffee maker – check. 5) Watch the morning news while I wait for my first cup – check. Sounds pretty easy, if I say so myself. Hold on, it's been twenty minutes. Why isn't the coffee maker beeping to tell me it's done? A trip back into the kitchen finds that I forgot to press the start button.

> **Be aware of each situation and consider the next step.**

What does that tell me? It tells me to be aware of each situation and consider the next step. If I think before I leap, most chores or events will keep me moving forward.

I think my short-term memory is a lot better now than it was during my first ten post-injury years, but darn it, short-term memory can make any day a less-than-good day. Plus, daily living is not just a memory issue.

It's way too easy to get distracted or fatigued, and short-term memory loss always seems to be waiting for an entrance. It's not a senior moment, it's a live and learn moment. Do I have to write a step-by-step process for everything I'm doing and glue it to my forehead? No, of course not. Instead of writing every step-by-step, I write and leave post-it notes in a conspicuous area where the "action" will take place.

When I'm going to heat up a can of soup on the stove or microwave, I have a timer in-between both appliances, along with a note taped next to the burner controls (on both the stove and microwave), telling me to turn on the timer. It doesn't matter why I turned the burner on; I have to turn the timer on before I leave and make sure the alarm is as loud as possible, so I'll hear it in a different room, even in the basement.

Let me give another example why I use a timer now. One time, I needed to make hard-boiled eggs. That's easy. Fill the pot with water, place eggs in the pot, turn on the burner, fifteen minutes later, turn off the burner and let the eggs cool.

> " I think my short-term memory is a lot better now than it was during my first ten post-injury years. "

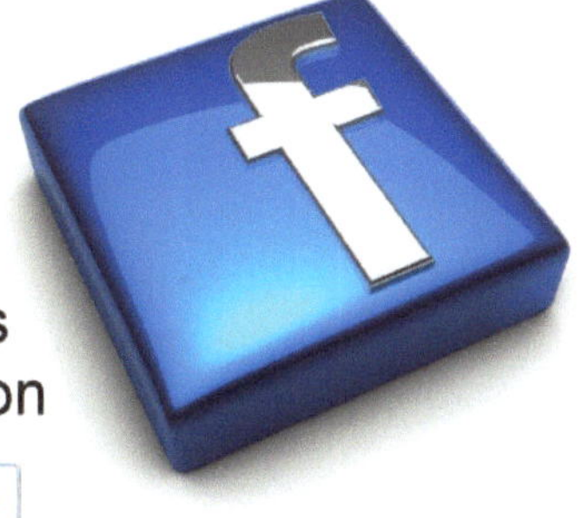

Join our Facebook Family

What do over 25,000 people from over 40 countries and five continents all have in common? They are all members of our vibrant Facebook family at /TBIHopeandInspiration

Well, you can probably guess that I didn't walk back to the kitchen after fifteen minutes. In fact, I wasn't back in the kitchen until the pan was empty and the eggs (shells and all), were almost burned up. Fortunately, a kitchen or house fire was not the path I broke ground with.

I used to think it was unfortunate to have my notes visible for everyone in the house, including family or guests. I don't think my family even notices them anymore, but friends and guests do. If they ask about them, I tell them the notes are my life vest and hope that they never have a brain injury. My notes keep everyone aware of brain injuries, but most importantly, the notes make me think.

Yes, my injury was over thirteen years ago, so shouldn't I have done everything or thought of everything of, by now? I wish. As I said in the beginning, I'm breaking a new path nearly every day.

> **"We have all heard that the brain has plasticity, but if we don't use it, we will lose it."**

A new path could just be a "new" way instead of the "normal" way. Do you always put on pants with your right leg first, then your left leg?

To create a new path, put on pants with your left leg first, then the right leg; then use this "new path" when putting on and tying shoes. It's not super different, but it's different enough that it keeps me thinking. When I'm going to do some regular task, I try to remember how I did it the last time and do the opposite. Doing that also helps with short-term memory.

My new path is not just making things okay, but really to keep my brain rewiring itself. Instead of being stuck in the past, it allows me to move forward. We have all heard that the brain has plasticity, but if we don't use it, we will lose it.

I have many more years to go (hopefully), and would prefer living more good days than the alternative. Take care and live with purpose.

Meet Ric Johnson

Ric Johnson is a husband, father, grandfather and a traumatic brain injury survivor from just over 13 years.

Ric is also a member of the Speaker Bureau for the Minnesota Brain Injury Alliance, and facilitator for The Courage Kenny Brain Injury Support Group.

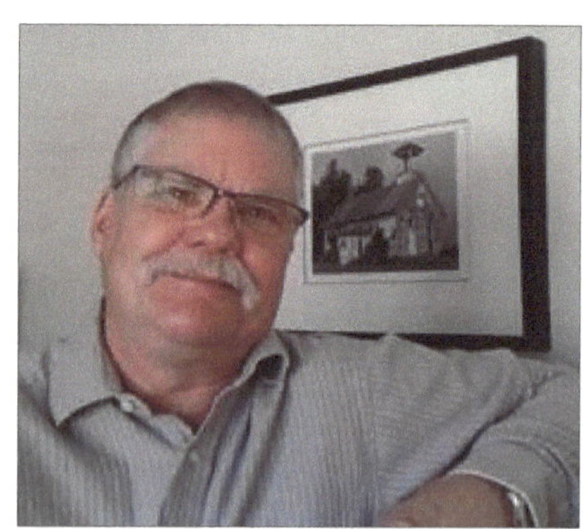

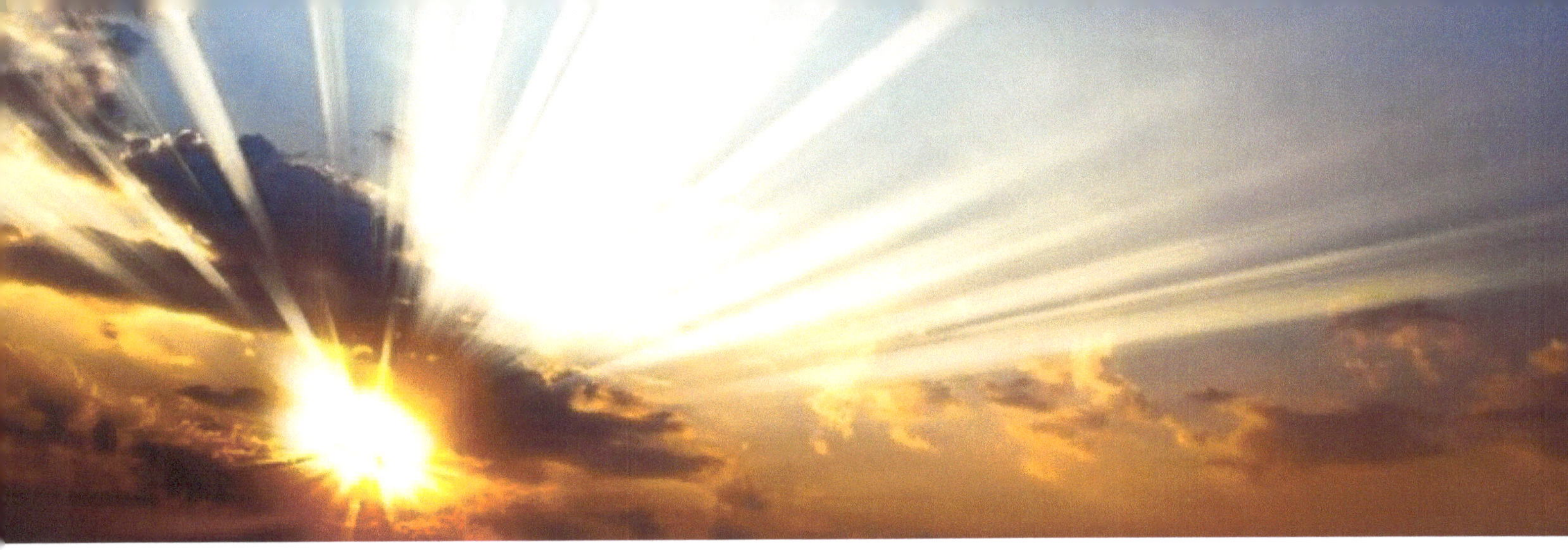

Love by Grace

By Kimberly Maronay

The past five years have been, by far, the most difficult of my life. When my husband, Chris, suffered his brain injury we had no idea what to expect. The hospital told us nothing. A couple of months after we were home, we received a package in the mail from The Brain Injury Association that explained everything. I finally had answers for why my husband no longer seemed like himself. The truth was, he wasn't the man I knew anymore. I had to say goodbye to that man and grieve the loss of a person who was still here in front of me every day. Now I had this new person in my life, and honestly, I didn't like him very much. My husband was kind to me, told me he loved me every day, and never would have raised a hand toward me.

This man, however, was cruel and violent. He was angry all the time. He knew no other emotion. How were we going to make it? I would not be afraid for my safety in my own home. I was not this woman. I had spent seventeen years with the love of my life; what was I to do now? He was still the man I married, the man I loved, the man I hoped to spend the rest of my life with.

We were already in separate bedrooms because we're both disabled, but this was not working. We needed to be under different roofs. Chris moved across town with our son, Cordell, and I fell apart. My whole world was crumbling around me. I didn't know how to be this version of us.

> **"I had spent seventeen years with the love of my life; what was I to do now?"**

We both showed up at each other's house almost every day. We Skyped and even shared family meals a few times a week. But, we were both not liking this new arrangement; it was not working for either of us. After one month, I had my guys back home. Still, it was a constant struggle trying to figure out how to get along and try to keep Chris calm and maybe find some peace. Even the doctors he tried to seek help from didn't know what to do for him, or how to treat him successfully.

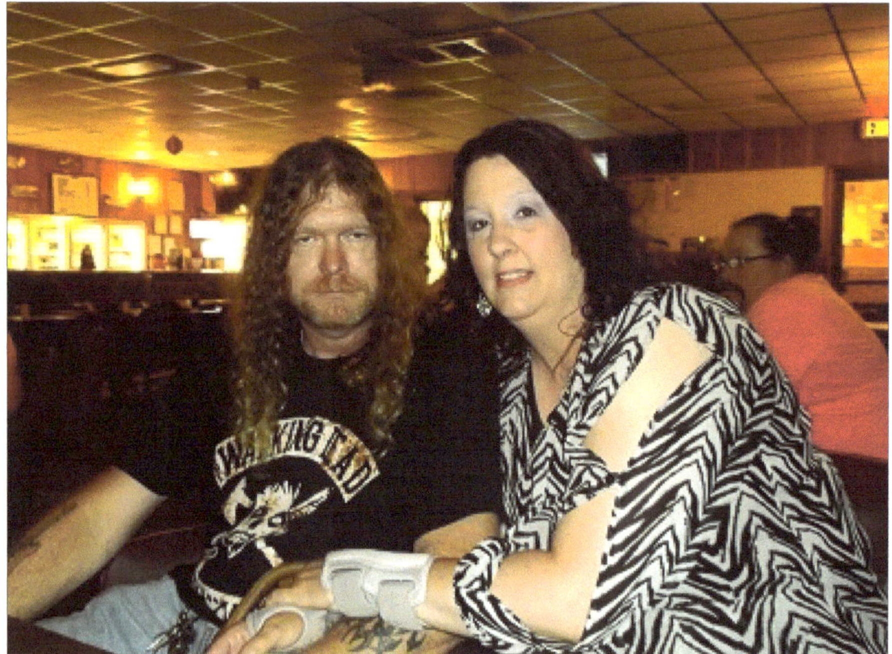

I had been praying for months, and it was the only thing holding me together. I thought about leaving many times, and I even kept a bag packed in my closet. Chris also threatened to leave on a regular basis. But, neither of us ever went through with it. We just were not willing to give up on our promises to each other.

We took our wedding vows very seriously and were determined to keep fighting. I began to pour myself into scripture and worked on my relationship with God. The movie "War Room" showed me a new way to pray, and I was very inspired. I began writing down scriptures and prayers and hung them all over my bedroom because I was at war. I was going to save my husband and save my marriage. Chris is resistant to trying anything, so it has to be my role. I looked at the life of Jesus and saw one constant thing: Love. I decided that no matter what I did or said to my husband, I had to make sure it came from a place of love.

I started noticing that while I was busy praying for my husband, I was changing. As I changed, he did too. We still had plenty of ups and downs, but things were slowly starting to improve. I began watching sermons on line and attending church locally again. One day it just hit me: when we were married, we became one. So whatever I do affects him and vice versa. All of my faith and prayers were having an effect on Chris as well as on me. I was feeling hope where I once felt defeated.

Living under one roof was still proving to be quite an issue, and we had to do something, but what? We were finally able to move Chris into the apartment right upstairs from our home. Now we had separate living quarters, separate bank accounts, separate bills, etc. Things were different, but we still worked together on everything. Being alone in a place to himself helped Chris to be calmer and more at peace. He was still angry all the time, but I began to notice him smiling once in a while! There were times where I know I saw the old Chris. Oh, how I still miss him. But this new Chris, well, I am starting to like him more and more.

We have had this living arrangement for several months now, and things are better than they have been since his injury. We still struggle every day because there is always some challenge. We are both completely committed to each other, and neither of us will let go of the other. We are here, together, always. I know that both my husband and my marriage were saved by love, and by the Grace of God. For Love endures all things, it is the greatest gift God has given us. If you love with all your heart, put your faith in God and never give up hope. Amazing things can happen. I have watched my husband change right before my eyes. One moment I saw a wild enraged man exploding in front of me, then in the blink of an eye I saw my dear husband once again calm and concerned. Miracles do happen. Chris may no longer be able to love me the way he used to, but that's okay. I can love enough for both of us. I can hope enough, believe enough, and pray enough for us both. Love and Grace. That is what saved us. We still have a lot of progress to make, but I have no doubt we will get there.

Meet Kimberly Maronay

Kim has been married for twenty-two years to her husband Chris. They live in Southeast Missouri, a rural area where very little is known about TBI even among the medical professionals. Kim has been disabled for ten years now, but still does the best she can to take care of her family. The struggles she has faced with her husband has brought her to know her purpose: to love this one simple man, unconditionally, for the rest of her life. She hopes to show others that with love and the Grace of God anything is possible, never give up hope.

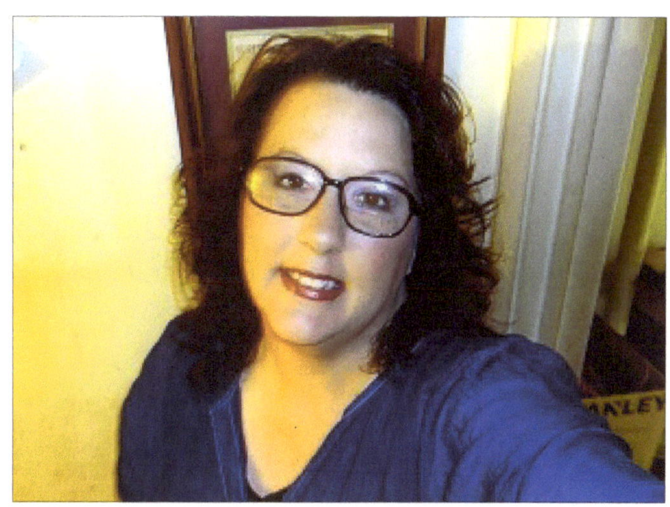

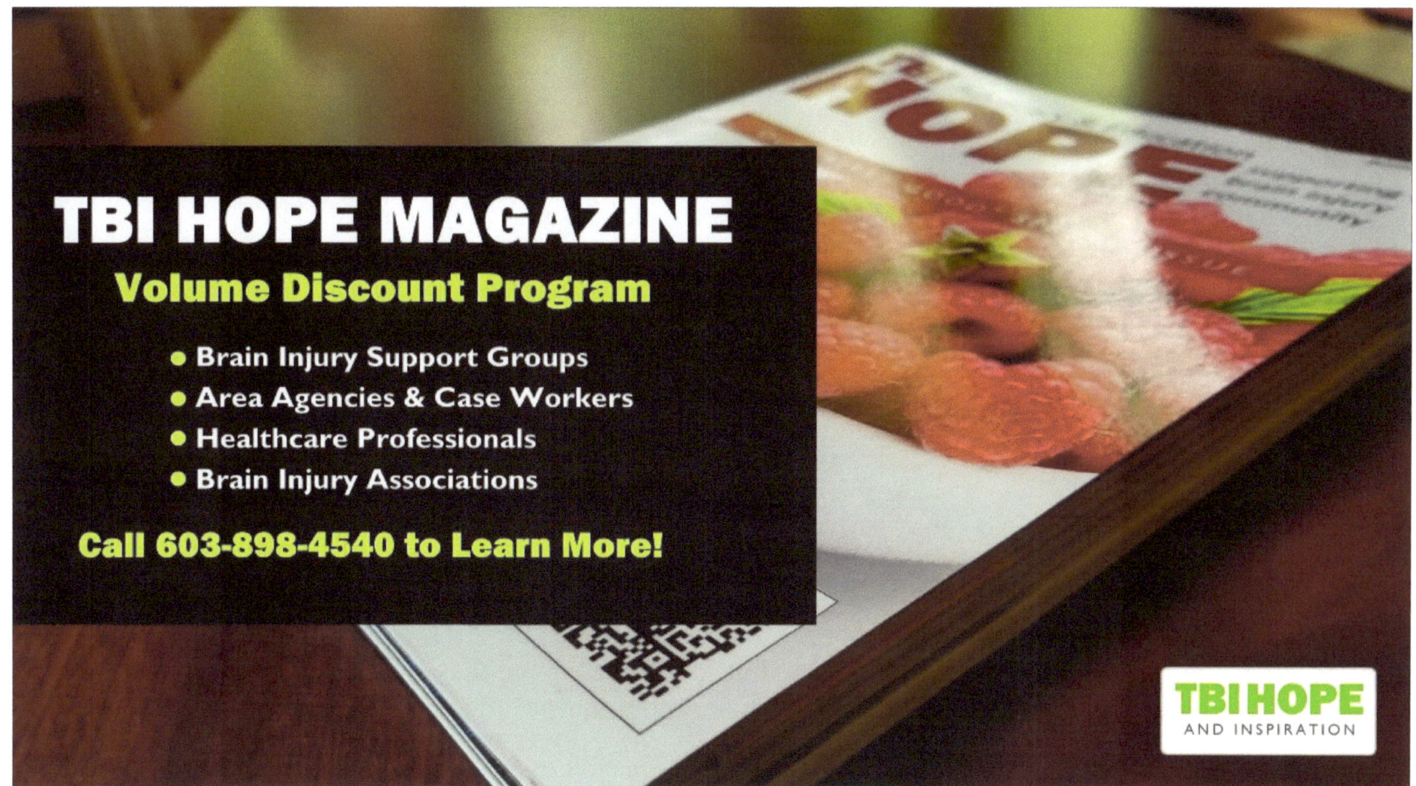

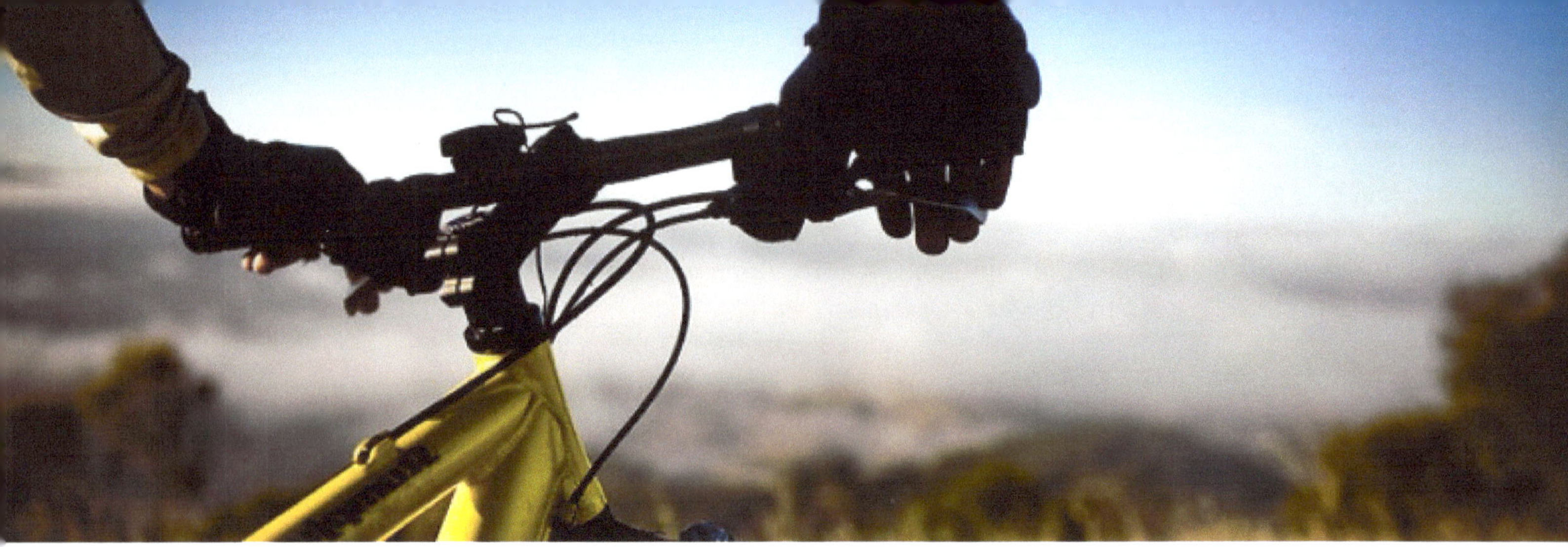

Look Where You Want to Go

By Rosemary Rawlins

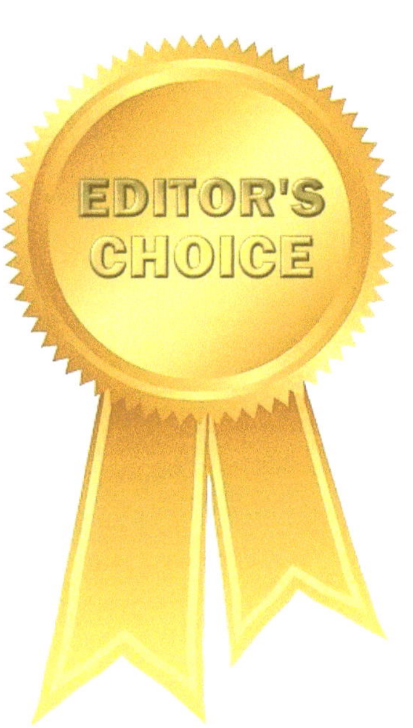

I wasn't always so fearful. There was a time when I felt secure in the world when I thought I had control over my own destiny. That time ended on April 13, 2002.

Before then, I didn't know that one moment could change the course of many lives, or that a hard knock on the head could erase precious memories or alter a person's personality. That our brain alone programs who we are by speeding up or slowing down our mental power, determining our behavior, and how well our body functions in the world.

I used to think the heart was in charge. I was a romantic. It was the brain all along. The brain alone can stop the heart.

Since the day my husband's head smacked the hard pavement after a fast car hit him, I've worked long and hard to let go of fear. Just yesterday, as Hugh drove me along Interstate 64 in a downpour, my right foot pressed into the floor hard enough to cramp my thigh when another car cut us off. I stopped breathing when the car hesitated for a moment as my husband hit the brakes. As I lurched forward, I saw myself fly through the windshield like I have a thousand times since the day he was hit. It's not only the crash that haunts me. My deepest fear lies in knowing the months and years of devastation that can follow one horrific split second.

"When you feel desperate, please keep looking until you can see beyond the wreckage of that one moment in time."

Because of my book and work on BrainLine.org, many caregivers contact me personally about their unrelenting fear of the future. Many say they keep reliving the day their loved one almost died. They are relieved when I suggest they may have secondary stress—something concrete with a name. A caregiver's personality can change pretty drastically and understandably after he or she witnesses a loved one's brush with death. Secondary stress might look like insomnia and hypervigilance or the inability to separate from a loved one's pain. A caregiver might morph from a relatively carefree person into an anxiety-ridden, overprotective, and controlling person.

We read articles all the time with headlines like: "Ten Tips for a Better Life" or, "How to Stop Stressing for Good." But the truth is, getting over the life-changing injury of a loved one is impossible—we don't get over it, but we can learn to live with it and find peace and meaning for ourselves. This healing requires a commitment to our own neglected health, visits to the doctor, following orders, and counseling. We need to take the medicine we are so used to giving! I know because it took me fifteen months to figure this out, and even then, I wasn't really taking care of myself—I was putting out fires. I would say, "It's time I slow down and make time for myself," but I didn't always do it. I made excuses.

I didn't realize that I had to stop seeing the accident everywhere I looked before I could see the life that was going on around me. My husband, Hugh, once coached a mountain biker, "Look where you want to go. If you look at the tree, you'll hit the tree." I kept looking at the accident as if I could find a way to rewind it, to undo it, to figure it out. It loomed like an obstacle I could not get around.

When I got sick and tired of being me, of feeling angry, bitter, sad, sleepless, and worried all the time, I searched day and night for a space between the trees where the sunlight found a path, and one day it was there. I walked away from one life and created another. When you feel desperate, please keep looking until you can see beyond the wreckage of that one moment in time. Because when you do, you'll create an opening in your life where you can begin to live and like yourself again.

Meet Rosemary Rawlins

Rosemary is the author of Learning by Accident, A Caregiver's True Story of Fear, Family, and Hope. She is also Editor of BrainLine blogs and a national speaker on caregiving topics.

You can learn more about her at:
www.rosemaryrawlins.com

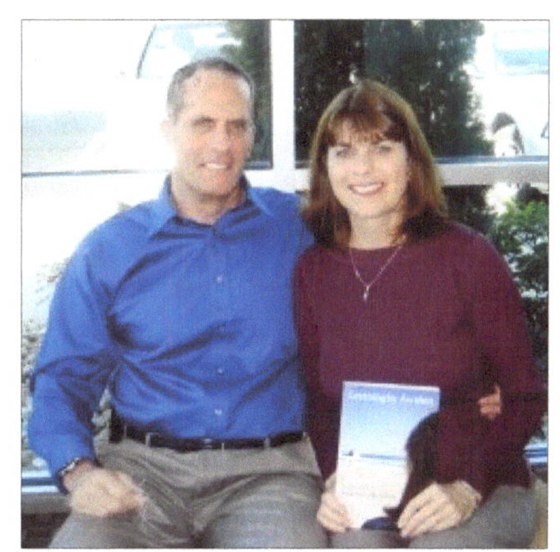

TBI HOPE Magazine
Photo Contest Winners!

Congratulations to our 2017 photo contest winners.
All winners will receive a printed copy of TBI HOPE
Magazine with their winning picture!

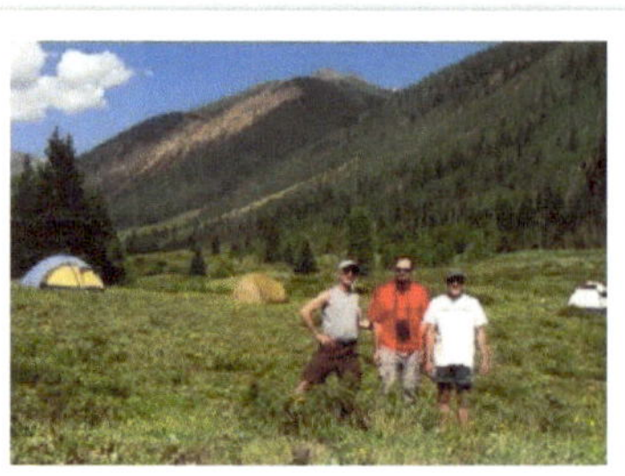

~Scott L.

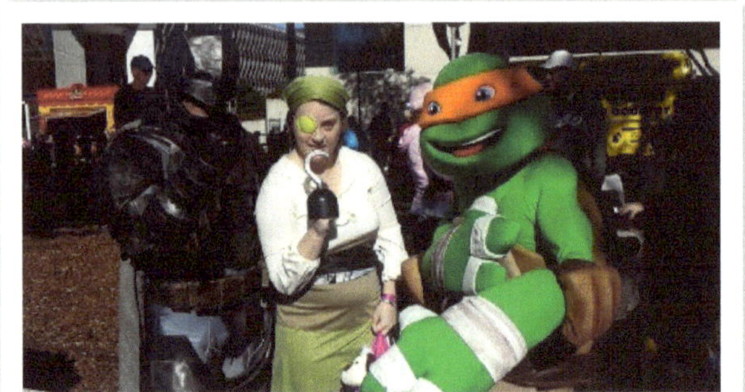

~Shannon B.

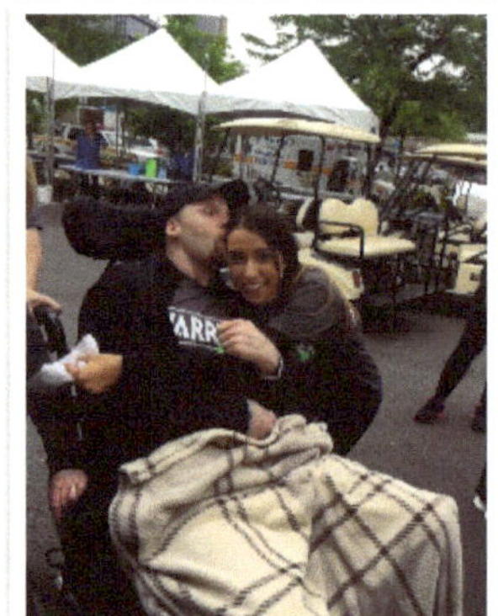

~Alyssa D.

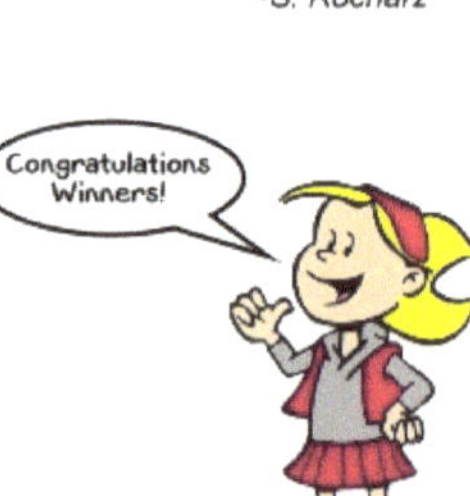

~S. Rocharz

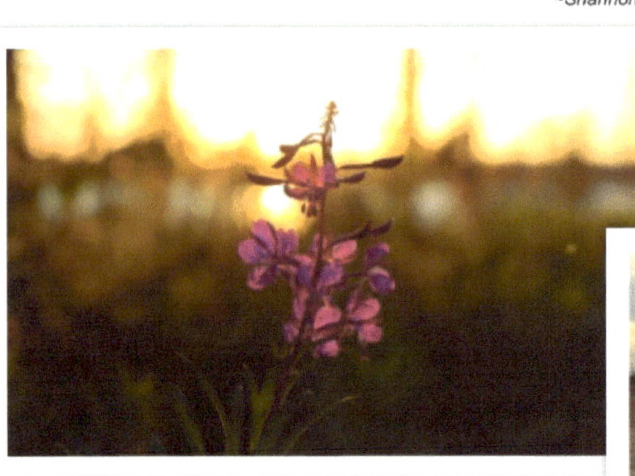

~Christa L.

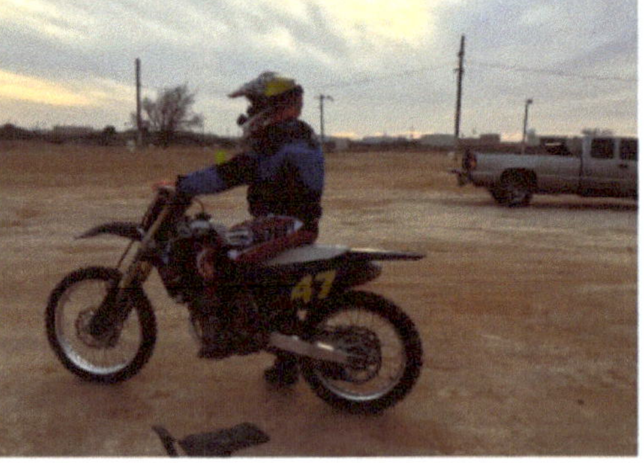

~Jenna E.

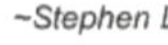

~Tiffany L.

~Stephen L.

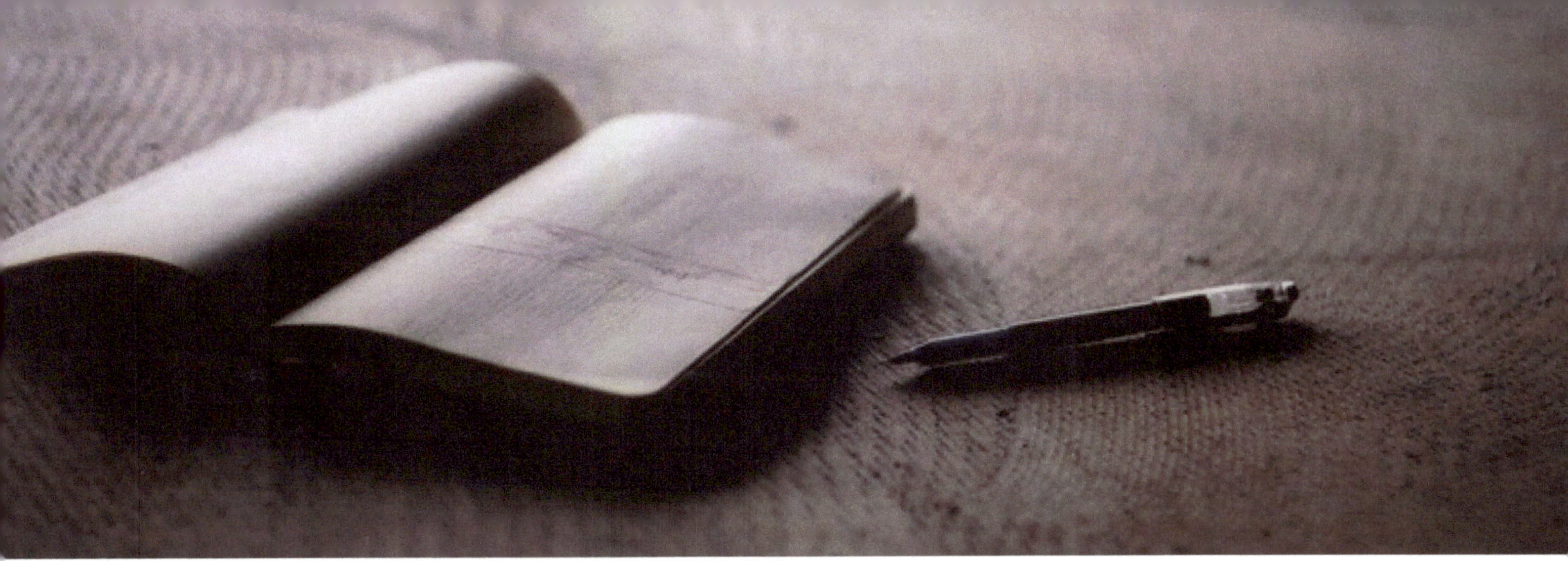

Against All Odds

By Laura Chagnon

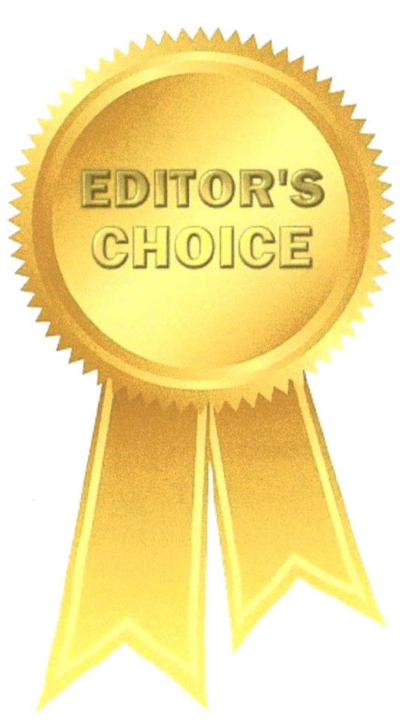

My name is Laura Chagnon. I am a TBI survivor and quite lucky to be here today writing this. I'm not typing this with my own hands; I need the help of others to do any physical tasks.

I'm 51 years old, and my life started off in good health. My major problem growing up as an adolescent was shyness. It was difficult mixing in socially at school, and I was bullied every day. During lunch in the cafeteria, I would be the only student sitting alone because I was like that puzzle piece that just didn't fit. It caused a lot of loneliness and frustration. Therefore, I needed to vent all of my built-up emotion.

English was my strongest subject in school. I enjoyed writing, so I began writing poetry. Never did I realize how my situation at this stage of my life would be so important later on. Ironically, those dark days would open up new doors later down the road.

I completed high school, despite all the bullying, but my self-esteem was left tormented. My life needed direction to become a stronger person. So, I chose to enter the military – the U.S. Army to be exact. I'm a very patriotic individual, so this venture seemed to be a perfect fit. My bags were packed, and my destination was Fort Jackson, South Carolina. Basic training, here I come. There was one slight problem. I always suffered from insomnia.

One day, my job was to carry a line of cable through the woods. I had gone days without being able to sleep and was utterly exhausted. So, I dropped the cable in the woods and went back to my barracks and collapsed. The drill instructor found me there and doctors realized continuing with basic training could lead to more serious health issues. I was given a medical discharge and sent back home.

I had to decide what my next path in life would be, so college seemed to be a logical choice. Soon I was enrolled in Springfield Technical Community College. I wanted to become a medical assistant. Everything was going in a positive direction. My grades were good, and I was excited. At 25-years-old, I could see myself graduating soon, getting a job and an apartment. Being independent would be a dream come true. My twenty-sixth birthday was fast approaching, and November 4th, 1989 turned out to be a life-changing day.

My mom bought me a gray suede jacket and a white leather pocketbook. I always did things spontaneously, and this day was no different. I took off and went to Boston on my own, driven by excitement with this adventure. In Boston, I decided to go window shopping and see the sights. Being a college student, there really wasn't very much money to spend, but I didn't care.

This fated November day started off sunny, but soon I was entangled by the dark shadows of that fall day in New England. It turned out to be the most traumatic nightmare in my life. I felt a tug on my new white purse that was strapped over my shoulder. Immediately, red flags went up, and I envisioned being robbed. Since I didn't have very much money, being robbed wouldn't be the worst thing that could happen.

I got spun around, and I stared into the eyes of two men. In a matter of moments, my life changed forever. My memory of the incident is very scarce. They brought me to a secluded area, and I don't remember what occurred since they fractured my skull. The assailants left my crumpled body on the streets of Boston to die and left the scene, never to be caught. Boston police found me and thought my gift of life was stolen.

However, someone was holding my hand and not allowing me to die. That was God, I suffered terrible injuries, but He had a path for me. It's ironic how at different stages of my life, I was trying to create a path. God intervened and set the right one before me.

My body was broken, and now I was a legally blind quadriplegic with a traumatic brain injury. Doctors gave me little chance of regaining much of my former cognitive ability. Was I going to give up on life? No way, my ever-loving God allowed me to live, and my goal was to realize he was opening a new door for me, even though it would take me more than four years to even see it. I went through physical, occupational, and speech therapy at various rehab centers. Finally, in 1992, I was able to return to live with my parents.

What would I do with my new life? I couldn't work a standard job with my physical skills being stripped. I needed caregivers 24/7. I guess I was in a predicament or was I? Remembering back to those adolescent years, I enjoyed writing poetry. Guess what? Now I had the time to delve back into that with a vengeance.

My process was dictating to my caregivers, and they would write down the words. When a poem was completed, it would be saved on my computer. I did this day after day, even submitting some of my works to local publications. A writer for the local newspaper even did an article on me in his human interest column and entitled it "In Poetry She Finds a New Spirit." I was excited and kept on writing with the goal of allowing others to read my words. Perhaps I could even publish a book. But that seemed to be quite a lofty goal.

Then in 2013, I met an angel. He was a short, stocky man who wore glasses. Perhaps not your typical angel – his halo was a bit askew. His name is Todd Civin. My soul mate had purchased a book that Todd co-wrote. We contacted Todd with the idea he would be able to bring a sampling of my poems to his publishing company and have them evaluated. We met for lunch and had a pleasant conversation. I explained to him my story and my dreams of becoming a published poet. I gave him about 20 of my poems to bring back to his publishing company. He said he would give us a call in about a week. A week went by and we didn't receive that much-awaited phone call.

My life had been full of disappointments up to now, and this seemed no different. Then, two weeks later, I heard the phone

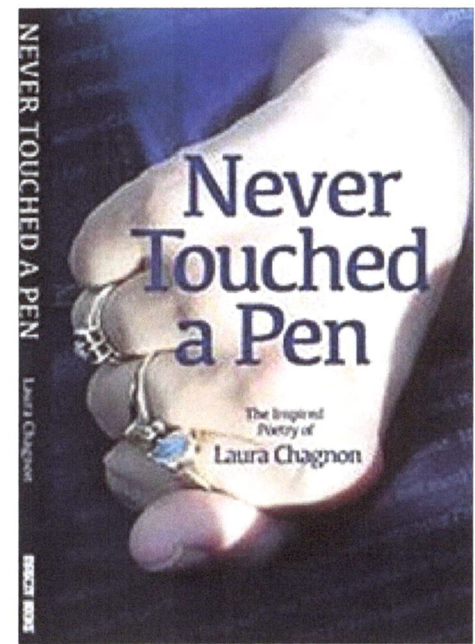

ring. "Hello Laura, this is Todd Civin from Mascot Books. Well, your story is quite incredible, and we think your poetry is amazing. The public needs to know about you and read your beautiful words. We would like to publish a book of your inspiring poetry."

At last a long-awaited dream come true! In April of 2014, "'Never Touched a Pen,' the inspired poetry of Laura Chagnon" was released. It was 25 years after my accident and I found out that dreams do come true. I am proud to say that I am a traumatic brain injury survivor and I continue to strive each day with God by my side.

Meet Laura Chagnon

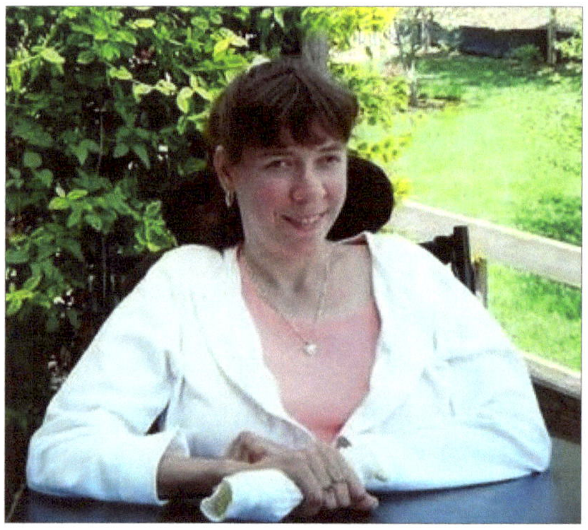

In 1989, on Laura's 26th birthday, she was the victim of a senseless assault in Boston, MA. She was left for dead in front of New England Medical Center where the assailant threw her out of his car. Doctors had given her little hope of being a productive member of society. This was all the fuel she needed to prove them wrong.

Laura Chagnon continues to craft poetry each day with plans on publishing her second book of poetry. Laura's book is available on Barnes & Noble.

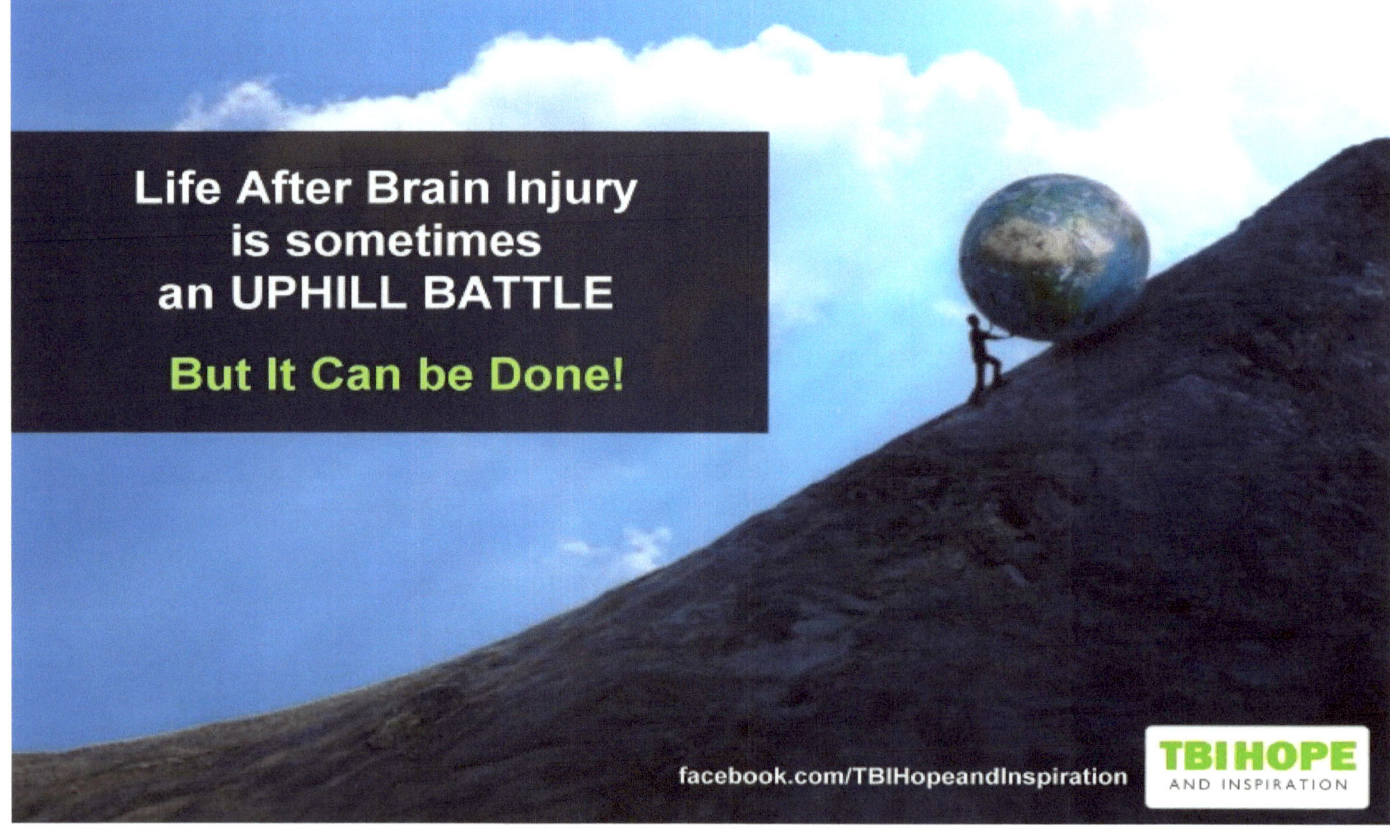

Self-Reinvention after Brain Injury

By Rodney Smith

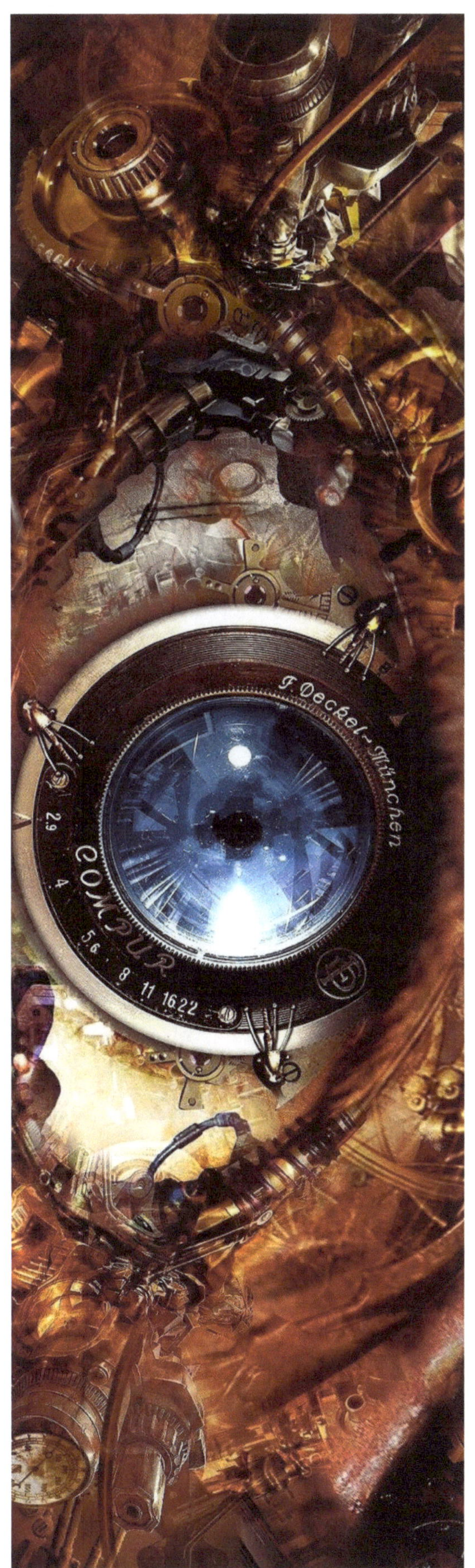

At some point adjustment occurs during the brain injury recovery journey, and there usually is an "a-ha" moment, if you will, where we realize that big and small changes have taken place. It is time to make the best of things as they are. Some of us look at this as "acceptance" or "adjustment," which is viewed by most experts as the final step in the grieving process. I don't know about all that. But, although it was hard to accept, I knew I had to change some things in my life after the TBI. Some of the changes were necessary because of deficits caused by the injury. Others were more personal and the result of a shift in priorities.

Before my TBI accident, I was a computer network engineer working on large, sophisticated, government systems. Afterwards, the skills weren't gone, yet, I couldn't process information fast enough to efficiently do the tasks my job demanded. Following several trips to my office, and a few attempts at studying material required for certifications in the field, I knew I would be a liability to my networking colleagues.

It is at that moment when I could have thrown my hands up and cried "Why Me?" However, God and Bonnie, my wife, wouldn't let me. Bonnie was persistent in pushing both me and the medical system to keep going. Looking back on that period now, she and I see how God was quietly and subtly directing our steps.

It took 2-1/2 months before we secured a referral to Shepherd Center, a private, not-for-profit hospital specializing in medical treatment, research and rehabilitation for people with spinal cord injury and brain injury. I received several evaluations and a recommendation for outpatient rehabilitation at Shepherd Pathways that included: a comprehensive community reentry day program, a residential program for patients ready to practice living in a more home-like setting, several programs and services available on an outpatient basis, and a short-term respite care program. That is where my reinvention began to take shape.

Before my accident, I had done some woodworking. It gave me a chance to do things with my hands, like my grandfather had always done. I saw and felt the products of my labor. As I started my occupational therapy (OT), my therapist asked, "What goals do you have?" One of the first things I chose was woodworking because I love to work with wood. But, I had to make sure I was capable of operating power tools.

My therapist and I spent a lot of time in OT sessions working on hand-eye coordination. I operated a powered jigsaw and a circular saw to see how well, and safely, I handled them. After I proved I was competent enough, I was given a project to build over a weekend. I made a simple recipe box, which I gave to my daughter Amy. We added the engraved label with her childhood nickname for humor. Through hard work, practice, and of course learning how to use new tools, my woodwork projects have gotten better. I have even made a couple of Christmas presents for the kids.

I know every TBI is unique with its own specific challenges. We survivors come from all kinds of circumstances and backgrounds and each individual has different goals, different skills, and different abilities. It is my prayer and hope that each survivor, regardless of his or her situation, who reads my story will be inspired to make the decision to keep moving forward, being the best that the TBI allows, and finding the open path to reinventing yourself, just as I was able to reinvent myself.

Meet Rodney Smith

Rodney's TBI happened on May 14th 2008 when a pickup truck failed to see him and crossed the road in front of his motorcycle. Before his accident, he worked as a network engineer on large complex government computer and email systems. As Rodney shares, "Life after a TBI involves continuous adjustment You are who you are so you have to make the best of the present." You can learn more about Rodney at www.hopeaftertbi.net.

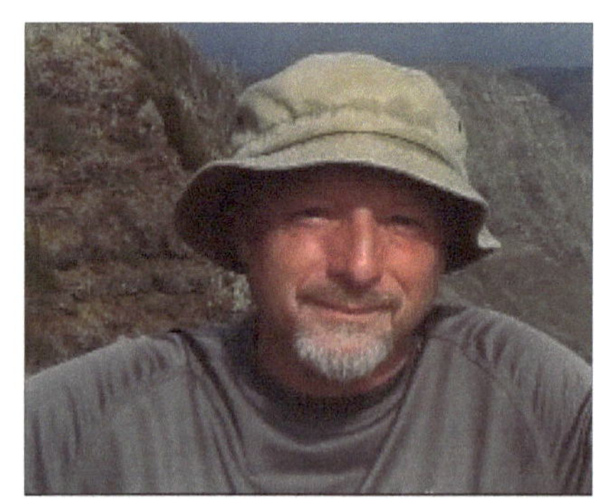

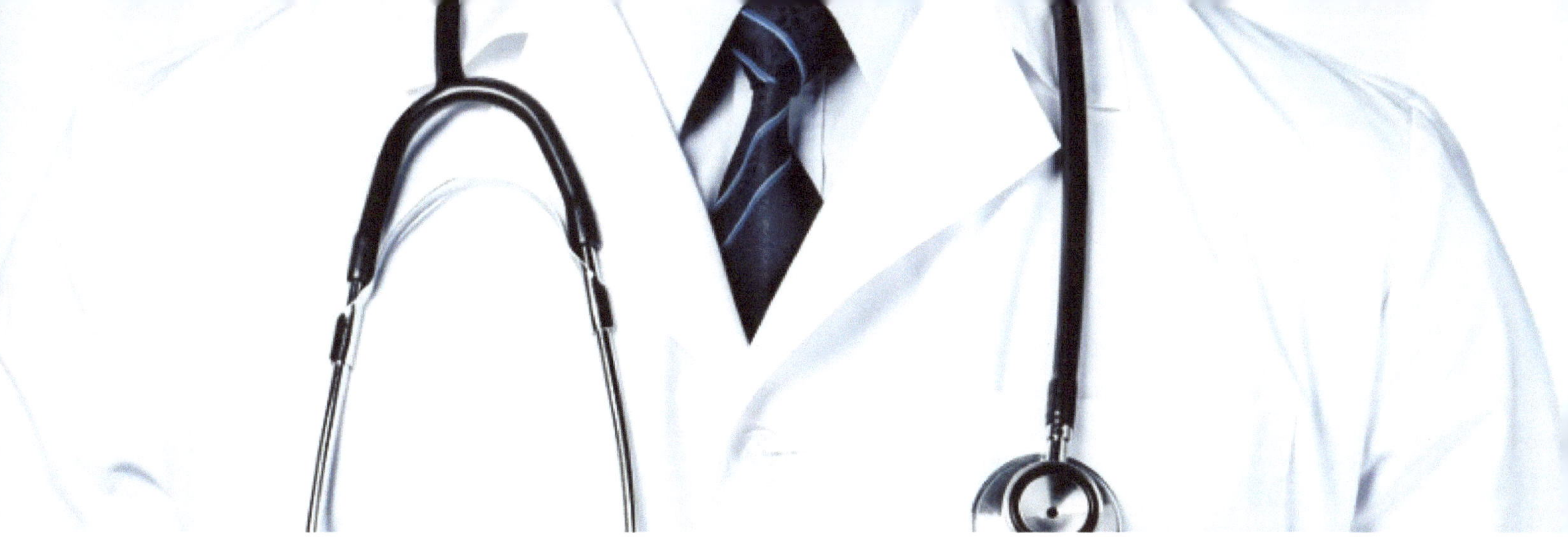

What Your Doctor Should Know

By Nancy Hueber

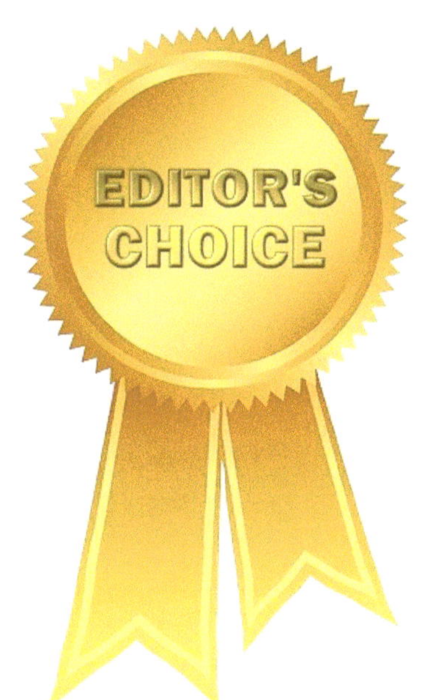

I am writing to you today because I will see you very soon for an appointment. Perhaps I just saw you, and the meeting didn't go so well for me. Maybe this list will help you with the next brain injured patient you see. Maybe your patients' files should all indicate whether or not there is a brain injury, as well as a hearing or vision impairment.

I think it's important to share where I am coming from before you step into the examination room, and what I have learned that works and doesn't work for me.

Ten Things Brain-Injured Patients Want Their Doctor to Know

1) I am a brain injury survivor. Therefore, there are things to consider about how best to conduct the appointment to make it truly beneficial for both of us. I will probably have someone with me if at all possible, to help me remember what went on, and how to help me at home regarding what was said.

2) Your fluorescent lights are going to trigger all kinds of bad stuff. Please understand I need to be wearing sunglasses or a cap, or both. If you can't turn them off, I'll try to remember my sunglasses! Maybe, if there are windows or a lamp in the room, we can just use that light while talking after the examination. I know you need the bright lights sometimes.

3) Please talk to me in softer tones, unless I happen to be hard of hearing. The brain injury has caused me to have light and sound sensitivity as time has passed.

4) Please don't be in a hurry to dispense a lot of information. Processing information coming at me too quickly is difficult. That is a newer development/deficit due to my brain injury and could be from the effect of medications. Simple, quiet questions are usually best.

5) Please write down whatever you find to be very important for me to remember. Or give me time as you are talking so I can write it down. It might be a longer appointment because of that, but it is the nature of brain injury. I may have memory impairment issues (short-term, specifically). In fact, if you ask me to repeat what you just said, you'll find out how well I grasped what you said. So, you might not want to use too many big medical school terms. I might even bring a voice recorder to help me remember what you said during our appointment. Thanks for understanding.

6) If I am in your office today because of pain, please don't talk to me for several minutes as we get started. Please listen, and don't rush to jump in. It's hard at times (especially when I'm tired) to compose and deliver my thoughts to you. On the flip side, please forgive me if I say them quickly and maybe frantically. I may be so overwhelmed by what I'm dealing with, and I may forget what I have to say if I don't let it all out in one fell swoop… and because it's been building up in me for two months or more since I scheduled this appointment.

7) Please do all you can to scope out my emotional well-being as we talk, and realize the daily difficulties of living with the results of a brain injury, along with the daily cocktail of medicines I've been inducing, perhaps for years. I may or may not be in need of anti-depressants, but I will surely be depressed if my doctor gives no indication that he's interested in how all this is impacting me.

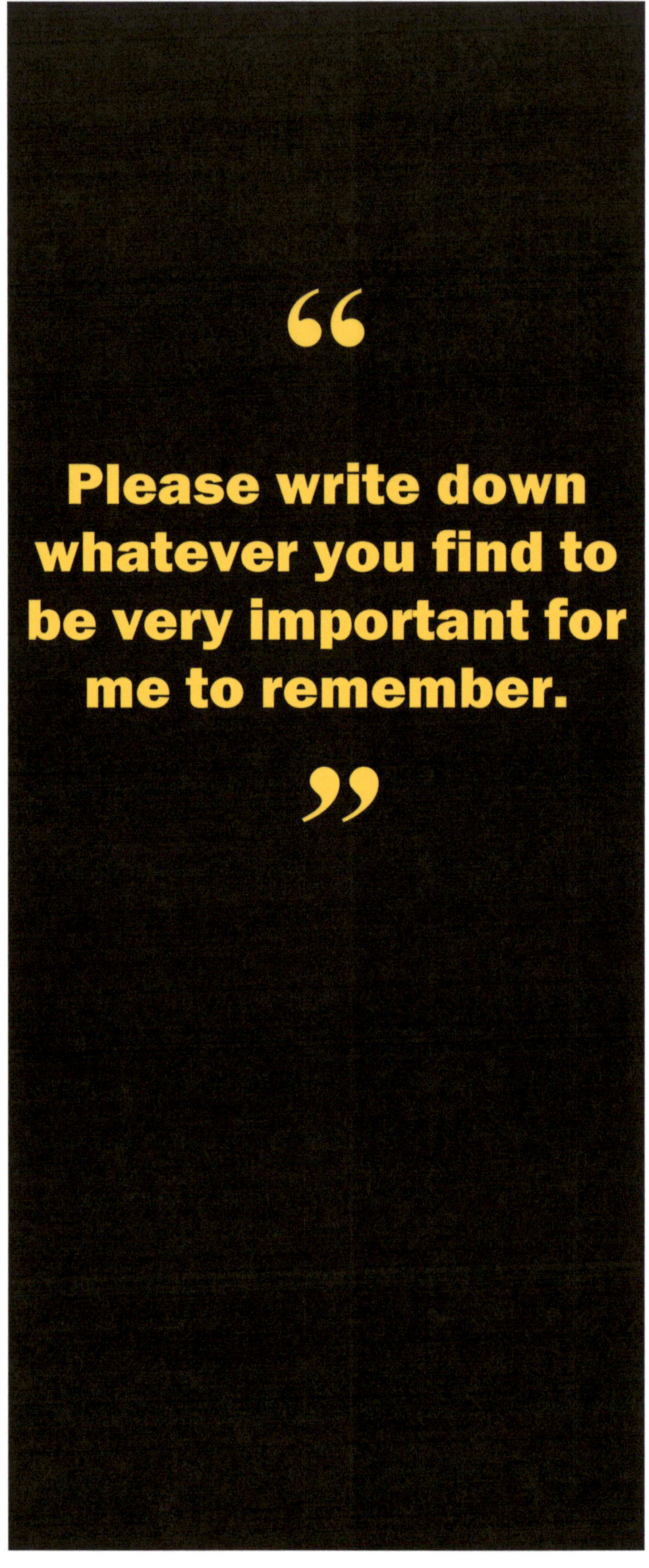

8) Please check on what I regularly eat by asking me. It's possible that my medicines and sickness are not the only culprits, besides my brain injury, responsible for my symptoms today.

9) Watch for physical cues that I'm getting fatigued as we talk. I might put my head on your desk or lie down on the table. I might cover my eyes or begin to look down. I might even get teary. You see, all of the talking and sharing of information has fatigued me to the point of mental exhaustion. The nature of the information has overwhelmed and maybe upset me. And to top it all off, I may have done other things - including traveling to the appointment - which has sapped my mental energy. It's amazing, the number of decisions my brain had to make before I stepped into your office or the visual and aural stimulations which may have already stressed my brain and emotions.

10) Please walk with me the short way back to the front desk (or have the nurse help me), so I don't have to remember how to retrace my steps. You'd be surprised how difficult that path back to the waiting room might be to someone who just shot their mental wad in your exam room. And if I had to come by myself today, I'm going to need all the help I can get.

Meet Nancy Hueber

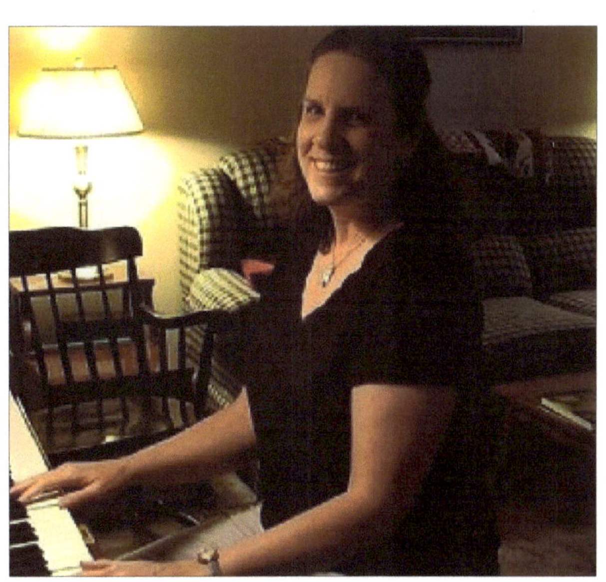

Nancy Hueber, a professional pianist, wife, mother, and frequent visitor to her couch and bed, survived a near baseball-sized brain tumor (meningioma) in the middle of her brain, and its removal by craniotomy six days later.

In 2012, Nancy and her husband Tom established a brain injury support group in their town in northeast Missouri, now affiliated with the Brain Injury Association of Missouri. Their monthly meetings average 20 attendees, both brain injury survivors and their caregivers, with injuries received from brain tumors, strokes, aneurysms, accidents and/or concussions.

I'm a survivor - a living example of what people can go through and survive.

~Elizabeth Taylor

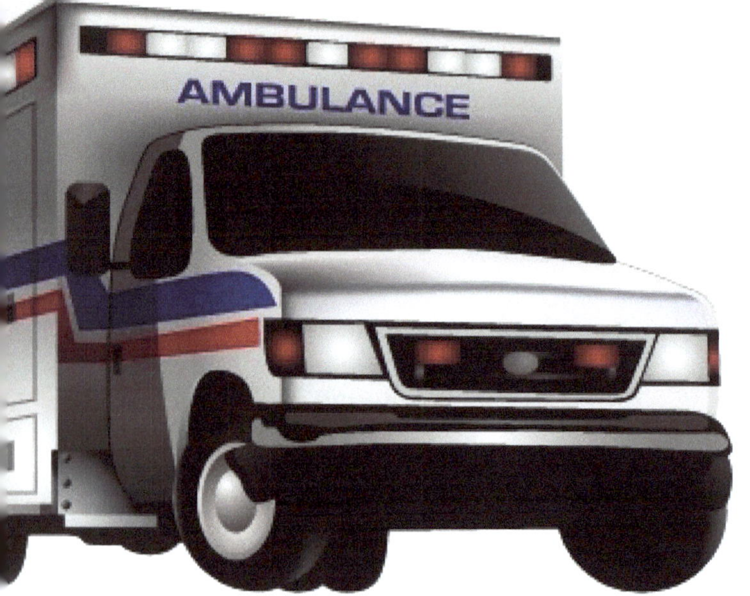
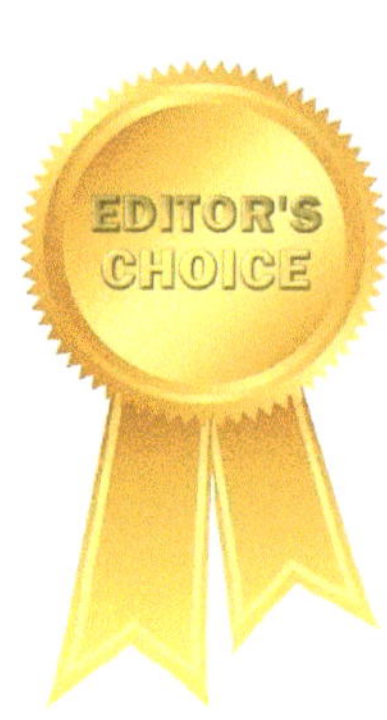

Miracles Happen

By Jennifer White

On July 28, 2000, I went from being an executive at a marketing company who serviced many national nonprofit organizations, to an unemployed housewife in a period of twenty-four hours. The cause: an intracerebral hemorrhage on my brain stem.

Living in a downtown apartment in Atlanta, GA, I lost consciousness and subsequently called 911. After speaking with an emergency operator who tried to calm me down by telling me I wasn't dying, I was rushed to a hospital via ambulance where I did die and was resuscitated en-route to the emergency room. I was intubated on the ride to the hospital and was admitted to the emergency room without brain stem reflexes.

The final diagnosis was severe coma in the presence of a massive interventricular hemorrhage. At the hospital, I had a right frontal ventriculostomy to eradicate the blood clot that sat on my brain stem and a sub occipital craniotomy to evacuate the hematoma and duraplasty. I then had a ventriculoperitoneal shunt performed.

The surgeon drilled a hole in my head to eradicate the blood that sat on my brain stem. My husband was told that I only had a 4% chance of survival. Following the surgeries, a feeding tube was placed. Due to the right lower lobe pneumonia, I was treated with multiple intravenous antibiotics. Six days later, the pneumonia started to clear and I was being weaned off of the ventilator that was keeping me alive.

As the pneumonia cleared and I started tolerating procedures more so than the days before, speech, occupational and physical therapy staff were asked to evaluate me for possible rehab. On the eighteenth hospital day, I was transferred from ICU to a bed on the hospital floor. On the twenty-fifth hospital day, I was moved to the acquired brain injury unit at a local rehab center where I was in stable condition but not out of the woods. I was in rehab for several months where I had to relearn how to walk, talk, eat, swallow, and perform simple tasks.

I also had to learn how to lean on others for help - one thing I was always too proud to do before the hemorrhage. Cognitively, I was a different person. I could no longer work and was placed on long term disability. I really wanted to work, however. I yearned for the day that I had to develop an annual marketing and budget plan for my clients or travel to a dozen different states pitching a new fundraising idea.

In a period of twenty-four hours, my future was determined for me. The days of easily navigating my life had ended with my traumatic brain injury. I now have to seriously think about every step I take, since my balance has been negatively impacted. My sequencing ability was seriously compromised and I frequently ask myself what goes first – socks or shoes? Shampoo or conditioner? I took everything that I knew prior to the brain injury for granted and had to relearn basic tasks that had taken me a lifetime to learn. I lost those skills in a matter of twenty-four hours.

What I never thought would happen actually happened. My fear of dying reared its ugly head when I was told I had died on the way to the hospital. The choice of whether I should have children was made for me when, after my brain injury, my surgeon recommended that I not have children. After the brain injury, I began to appreciate things more. I had a new perspective on my life and learned what true love is from the kindness I was shown by my family. My husband was so loyal and extremely committed to my survival. He forced me to get up when I just wanted to die. He helped me walk when I just wanted to give up. I try to thank him for his loyalty, but he is such a humble man he just asks me, "How could I not have helped you?" I also have siblings that helped me too. I'll never know entirely what my brain injury did to all of them. I think, however, we all grew some that day.

After the day of the brain injury and it was clear that I would live through the nightmare, I set off to recreate my life as someone who would more than likely never work again. I took classes to be a master gardener. I learned how to quilt, and have made at least twenty so far. I dedicated my mental energy into being the best wife ever and believe that it is my husband's time to shine.

"My success is no longer measured by how much money I make or what kind of position I hold at work."

Get Your Facts Straight: Kids & Concussions

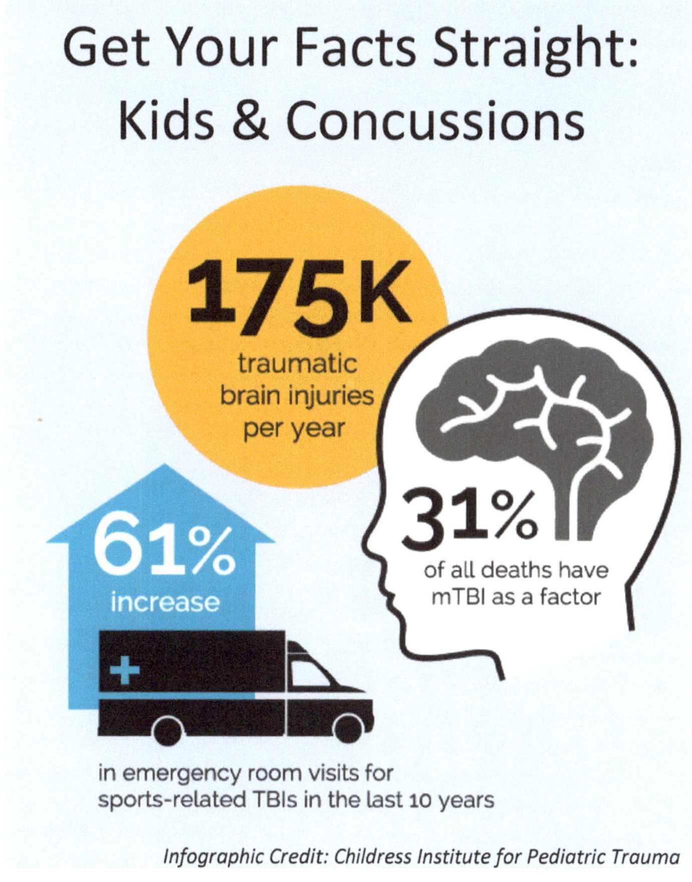

Infographic Credit: Childress Institute for Pediatric Trauma

It is his turn, and he is doing very well. I started seeing a new outlook on life. Colors are brighter, relationships are sweeter, and my success is no longer measured by how much money I make or what kind of position I hold at work. My success is measured by how kind I am to people and how much of myself I can give.

This is actually different than when I lived in downtown Atlanta in a high rise apartment and worked seven days a week. I do feel some survivor's remorse, but I am happy to be alive! The guilt I feel from putting my family through so much pain is starting to lessen a bit. It has given way to thankfulness for being alive. How many people get to do a "do-over" in life? It was the worst time and the best time because I did not die but was left with a question: How am I going to live the rest of my life? I am confident that I am most likely unrecognizable to those who knew me prior to the brain injury. Not physically, since I pretty much look the same, but emotionally. Rather, I am now a softer, kinder, less aggressive and more introspective person. And of course, I still deal with painful headaches, cognitive deficits, and balance issues. But, the number of good days are becoming greater than the bad ones. For this I am happy.

Meet Jennifer White

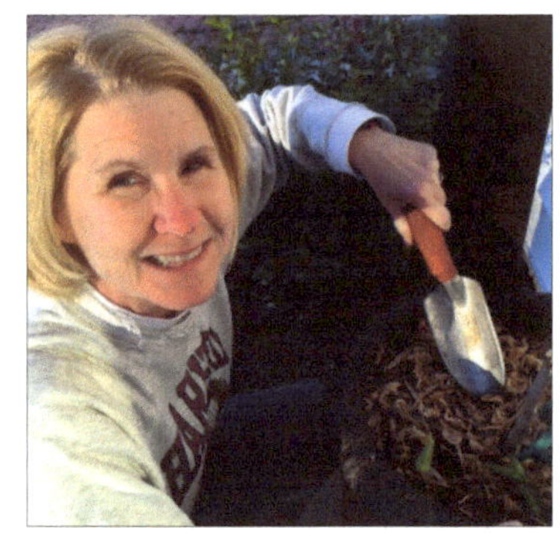

Jennifer White is a traumatic brain injury survivor from St. Louis, Missouri. When she's not writing about her life as a survivor, she enjoys spending time with her family and of course, quilting.

Living With Hope

By Patrick Brigham

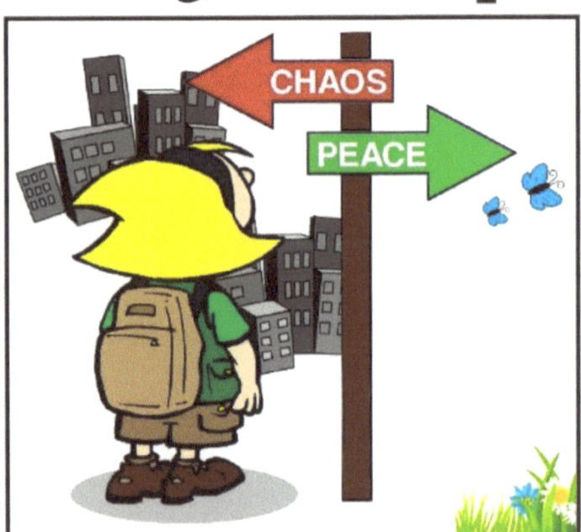

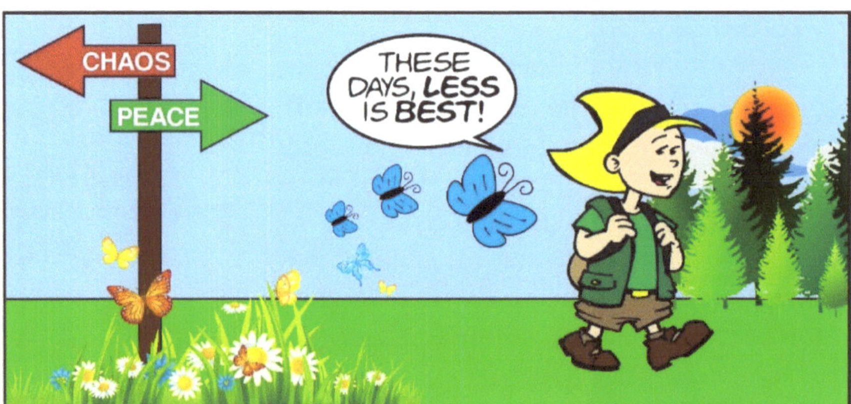

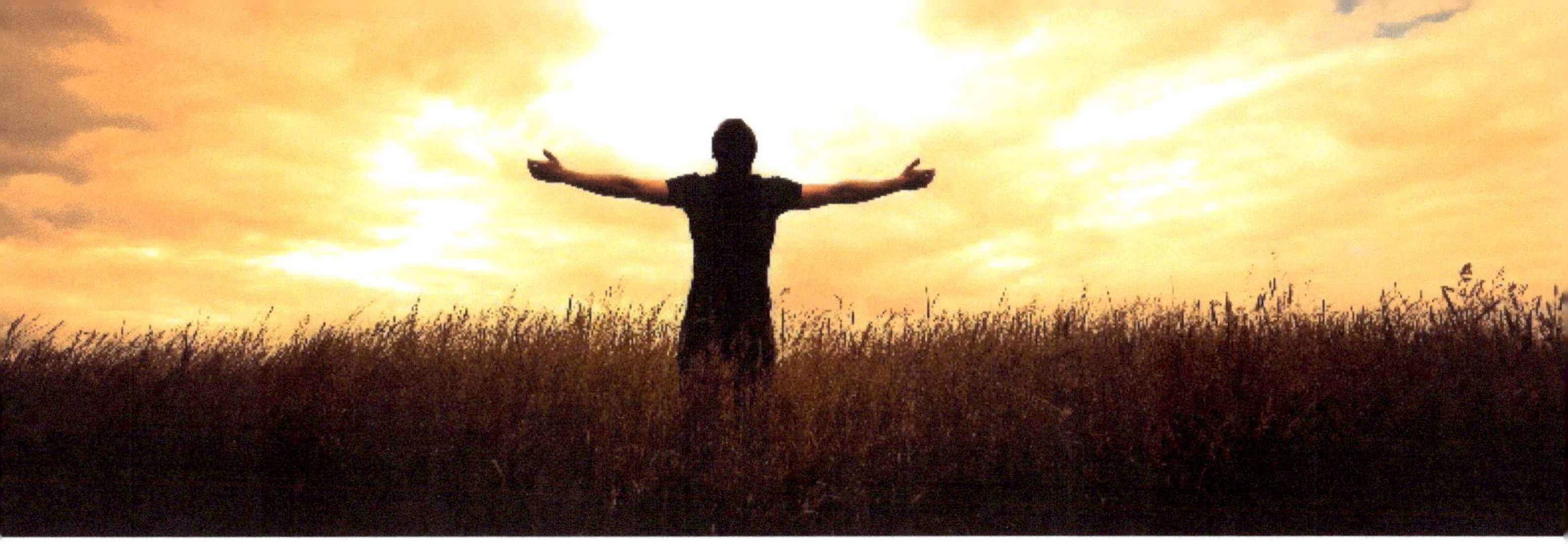

Creating Success in our Lives

By Jeff Sebell

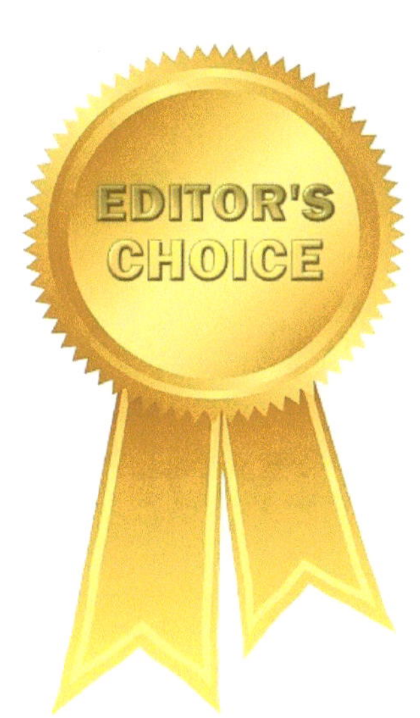

Life changes when you experience a brain injury: those of us who have experienced a TBI know this better than anyone else. Life becomes a crazy, mixed-up jumble, where everything has changed…except for one thing.

The one thing that doesn't seem to change is our expectations: our expectations about what we should be able to do, as well as how we should be able to function as human beings.

A brain injury is sudden and cataclysmic. After experiencing a TBI, we are forced to go through a learning period where we attempt to come to grips with the changes that have occurred. That takes time. There are so many changes that it can take years for us to understand all of our capabilities. Not until we know our capabilities, can we adjust our expectations.

Learning about ourselves and adjusting our expectations is crucial to creating success.

Many of us feel that changing our expectations is the same as throwing in the towel and giving up. Of course, no one wants to surrender, and we need to realize that changing our expectations is not the same as giving up. Rather, we are adapting to our new circumstances. We are learning what it takes to thrive in a new world.

Much of our self-worth and happiness is based on how we, as human beings, relate to and fulfill those expectations. When our capabilities change due to TBI and our expectations do not adjust, we are setting ourselves up for repeated failure. We become stuck in an old reality, and we continually beat ourselves up and get down on ourselves for not being able to do something we have always been able to do.

Some of the most debilitating effects of brain injury are these negative feelings that we develop about ourselves, and how these feelings and thoughts affect what we do. However, how we feel about ourselves is driven by our expectations, and thus, is something we can control.

Yes, while we may not be in complete control of our capabilities, we are in control of our expectations.

The equation is simple: To feel more successful I would need more successes, and to have more successes I'd have to change my expectation of what success is for me. I need to adjust, so I am not beating myself up so much.

Starting Anew

We spend years getting to know ourselves and creating expectations for ourselves. These expectations come naturally when we see how we function in situations, and we take pride in being able to perform and fulfill our expectations.

Anything that involves risk and change can be scary.

The knowledge we have gained over the years is thrown away in a split second by brain injury and rebuilding that knowledge base is difficult. No one wants to chuck aside all their life experiences, as well as all the work they have invested in themselves –the work that has created the expectations they have - and start anew.

Our pride is involved. Our ego is too. We find it difficult to give up what we knew about ourselves, but, the reality is we have changed, and we are asking our expectations, based on what we have learned about ourselves, to change. It is important to understand that creating a culture of success has less to do with what we do and more to do with our expectations.

We are facing some period of time where we are getting to know our new "selves." It's not always easy to adjust our expectations. We have to go through a lot of trials and failures in order to learn about ourselves. And you have to put your ego aside so that you can accept your new expectations.

If we don't adapt and learn we will be trapped in a cycle of failure. We want to build a culture of success, where we understand our capabilities, and we build our expectations around what is possible.

Finding a way to be successful in life after TBI is so essential. It can also be scary. Anything that involves risk and change can be scary. In fact, we may be even more comfortable keeping our old expectations, knowing we will continue to fail, rather than to take risks and try to be successful.

Changing your expectations doesn't mean giving up dreams and aspirations, but it may mean changing them or re-examining them to either make them come true, make some semblance of them come true, or make something else happen.

The goal here is not to beat ourselves up all the time, either for things we can't do that we think we should be able to or for ways that other people act towards us. The ultimate goal should be to feel satisfied and productive, and we can start by making a very personal choice to change the expectations we measure success against so they are realistic and attainable.

Meet Jeff Sebell

A long-time survivor, Jeff is the author of "Learning to Live with Yourself after Brain Injury." You can read more about Jeff and his journey on his blog at www.TBISurvivor.com

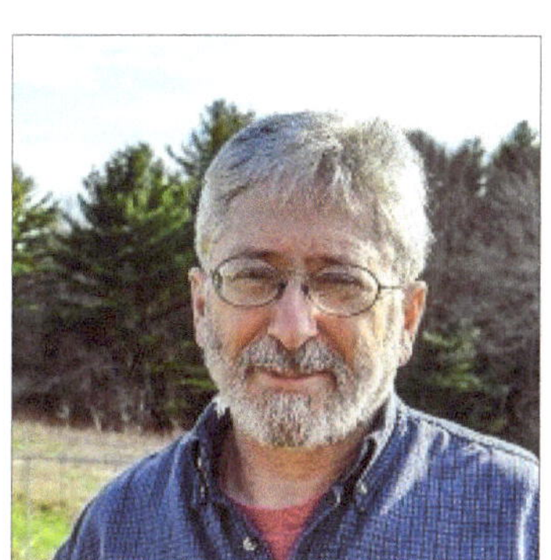

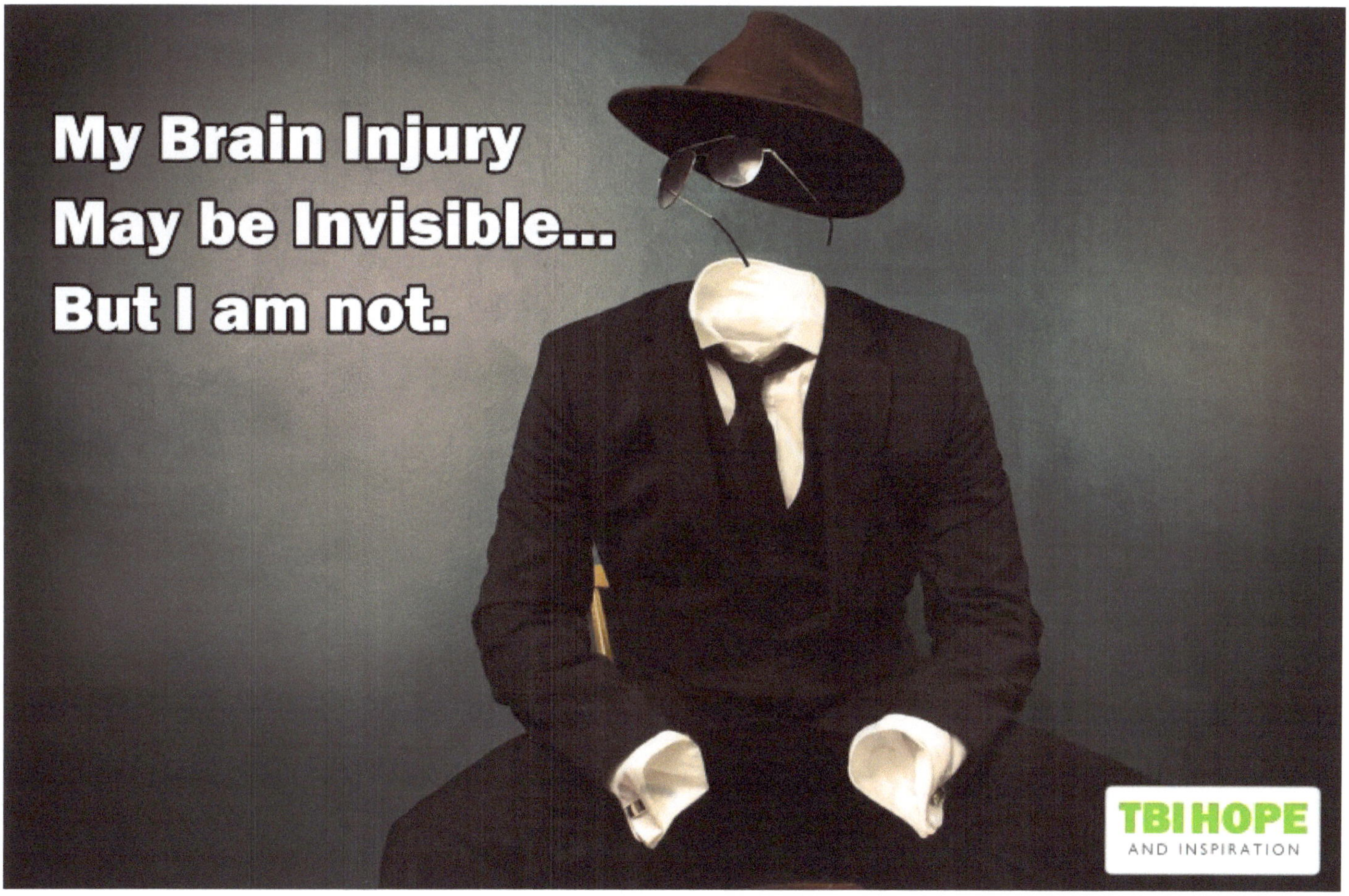

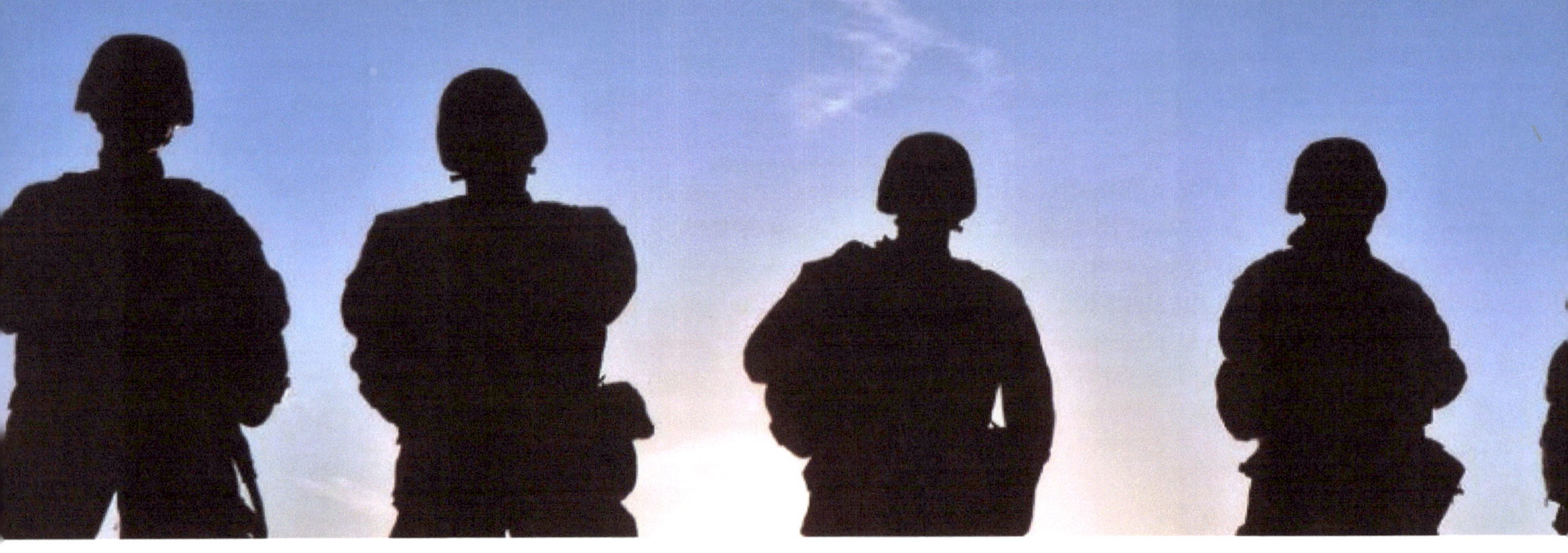

Is the VA Raising the Bar for Healthcare

By Karee White

As the largest integrated health care system in the country, our Veteran Health Administration (VHA), within the Department of Veterans Affairs (VA), serves nearly nine million Veterans each year. Wrought with problems and plagued by sharp criticisms, it is the entity whose mission is to care for that very special group of people who served our country, in both good and bad times. Rarely a day passes that a reader can't easily find a newly posted negative story involving the VA. It begs the question, is the VA caring for our Veterans or simply *managing* the care of our Veterans?

Yet, there is an emerging shift now occurring within the VA; one that speaks to the future in a way that may solve much of the unfilled, long-term care needs of our Veterans. It's called the Veteran-Directed Home and Community Based Services (VD-HCBS) Program, and it's giving our Veterans choices and control over how to meet their health care needs. "This program is taking our overall health care system to the next level, changing the very way we meet people's needs," said Lori Gerhard, Director, Office of Integrated Programs, Administration for Community Living. "The VA is very much focused on putting Veterans in charge of their care." VD-HCBS fits with Secretary Shulkin's goal of Veteran-centered care, by partnering with our Country's Nationwide Aging Disability Network to deliver the services that the Veteran needs. "States have developed long-term services and support over time, and it makes sense to use the expertise of these local agencies to assist Veterans in determining their care needs," Gerhard commented. "VA leadership is making the investment in helping Veterans design their care to fit their life; and they're more engaged in their community."

So, who are good candidates for this program? "Veterans and Caregivers who are interested in designing their own plan of care," said Dan Schoeps, Director, Geriatrics and LTC Purchasing, Veterans Health Administration, adding, "Maybe their needs are not being well met through traditional agency care." Indeed, Veterans that typically need more than twenty hours a week of help are at risk of placement in a nursing home.

The initiative shifts from provider-oriented care, to participant-directed or self-directed care. Simply put, the Veteran determines their needs with the help of a counselor from a local aging and disability network-contracted agency in their local community.

The counselor develops a budget for the Veteran, and the Veteran decides who and what services they want to pay for their needs. The Veteran can hire family or friends, using this budget. "I am more in control of who walks through my door and is injected into my family life. Indeed, being able to hire family members is a definite bonus," shared Lauri Rogers, who cares for her son David, a 28-year old Veteran who lives at her home, having suffered a Traumatic Brain Injury several years ago.

This latest VA initiative shows a firm commitment to expanding access of long-term services and supports for Veterans who require a nursing home level of care, but who desire to remain in their home and community.

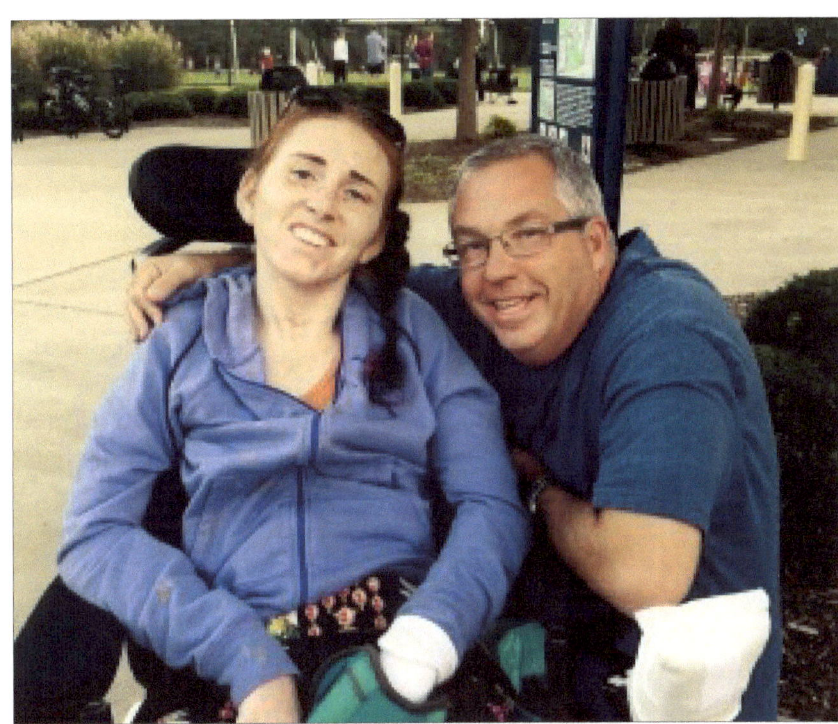

Captain (R) Kimberly Fix with her High School Tennis Coach

The self-directed movement isn't exactly new. In fact, its roots stem from 1996 when scholars like Boston College's Kevin Mahoney, Ph.D. drove research to propel participant or self-direction as an innovative model. It created a wave of new programs around the country, largely due to the extremely positive impact on participants, family caregivers, and even workers.

In 2008, he looked to the VA for a larger, more targeted audience. Mahoney's self-directed model led to a partnership between the VHA and the Administration for Community on Aging. No other agency knew long-term care better than the latter. And, the former presented a population that was compactly nestled within one hospital system. In 2015, under the helm of Secretary Bob MacDonald, Congress mandated legislation that targeted rebalancing VHA's long term care initiative, specifically addressing VD-HCBS. Money was set aside at the VA Central Office, to be used only for Veteran Choice Program initiatives, to include VD-HCBS. Using Veterans Choice dollars, an individual VA Medical Center (VAMC) contracts with a local Aging

Though many Veterans currently do not have access to Veteran Directed care, it is coming.

Disability Network Agency to assess and provide VA-targeted Veterans with a budget to choose community services and supports. But, like many good ideas, it advanced slowly in its eruption, with a rollout to just a handful of VAMC's which volunteered to pilot the program. When David Shulkin took over the helm as Secretary of the VA, he specifically mentioned the VD-HCBS Program, announcing that it will be in every VAMC within three years.

Currently, VD-HCBS is in 37 states, with 100 Aging Disability Networks assisting in the implementation of this program at the local levels. Largely due to Schoeps' efforts, the VA has created a standardized tool to develop each Veteran's budget, based on their local area costs, ensuring equitable distribution across the US in allocation, while expanding Veteran access to care as well. "The focus is 'Veteran-centric'," mentioned Schoeps. He emphasized the effort from the strategic partnership developed at the highest levels of government, implementing a structure downward to create a direct link at the local community level between the Veteran and the aging agency, the local experts in the community for helping disabled and aging find resources. Veterans should speak with their VAMC to see if they can participate in the program.

Though many Veterans currently do not have access to Veteran Directed care, it is coming. The VD-HCBS Program has grown by word-of-mouth. And, as interest continues, more VAMC's are meeting their certification requirements to administer the program in their area. Still, some Veterans feel the change isn't coming fast enough. There are even VAMC's with waiting lists, as is the case at San Diego's VAMC. Secretary Shulkin has directly committed to this program, and funding has been extended until the current budget dollars are expended, expected to last into early 2018.

Studies have shown remarkably positive results in the areas of individual Veteran satisfaction, and cost savings to the VA organization itself. In a recent, small study comparison of VD-HCBS to Community Nursing Home Placement, conducted by scholars of the Medical College of Wisconsin, living at home costs were just half the price of living in a Community Nursing Home. For twenty-five Veterans, the cost savings would amount to almost one million dollars per year to our VA. And, Veterans reported greater satisfaction and feelings of safety living at home, and being able to participate in their community.

The infrastructure of our current US Healthcare System is program-centered; provider-payer centered. Veterans, like in broader society, have received care from available resources and services. But, that's changing, and the VA's implementation of VD-HCBS may actually change the way our greater health care system meets people's needs. Perhaps, through this program initiative, the VA may ultimately raise the bar for the overall health care system in the U.S.

Meet Karee White

Karee Van Wert White served three tours of duty in Europe and the US, leaving the service as an Army Major, a paratrooper in Special Operations Command at Fort Bragg. White continued to embrace the fitness standards she loved in the military, training nationally as a Fitness Instructor to train others in her local community, while she and her husband of 30 years raised their nine children. She also wrote for several local newspapers in her community, advocating for the many achievements of community members. Three years ago, her oldest daughter suffered a Traumatic Brain Injury in an auto accident following combat deployment to Afghanistan. White spent the next year by her daughter's side, advocating and supporting her as she remained in a coma. Two years ago, the White's brought their daughter home to live with the family. As the mother of five military, White continues to pursue Veteran support initiatives.

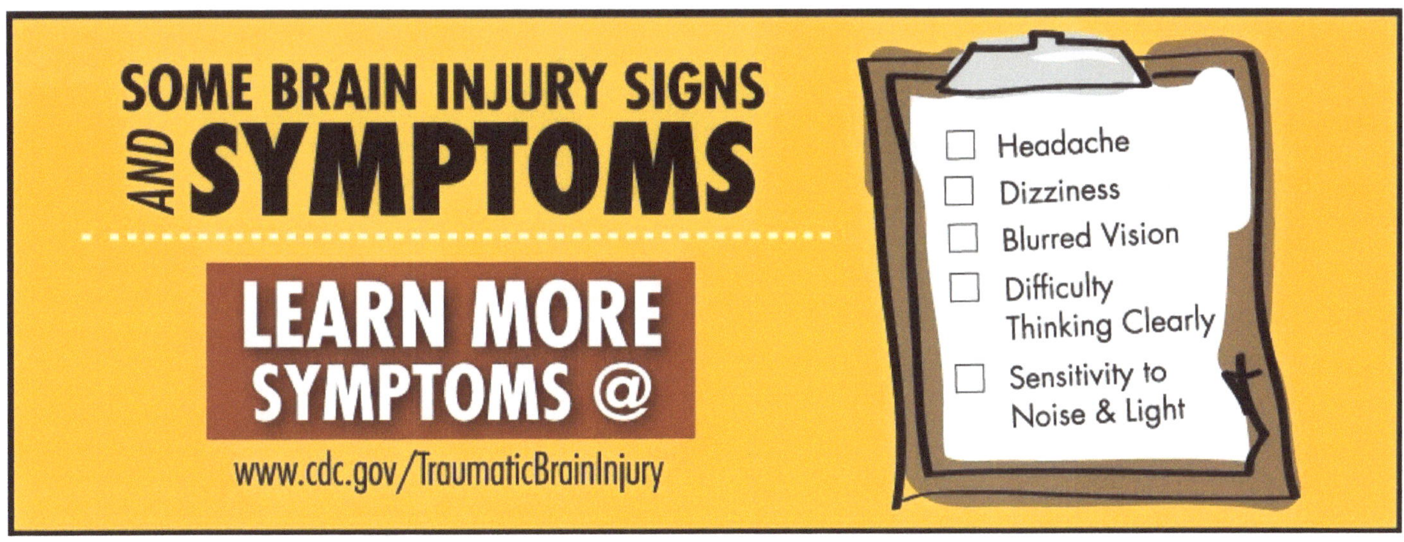

At the TBI HOPE Network, we are always looking for ways to advocate for those affected by brain injury. Our goal is to be as *inclusive* as possible. Though most people never noticed, there has been a slow and steady shift over the last year in how we speak about brain injury. Years ago, most all forward-facing references used the term *Traumatic Brain Injury.* But as time has passed, we realized that term was limiting. What about stroke survivors? How about those who have experienced an AVM or anoxic brain injury? We were unknowingly excluding thousands of people from much-needed support.

Earlier this year, I posted a note that always appears to first-time visitors to our Facebook community. It reads in part, *"Our group is open to ALL affected by brain injury. Those who have experienced a TBI,*

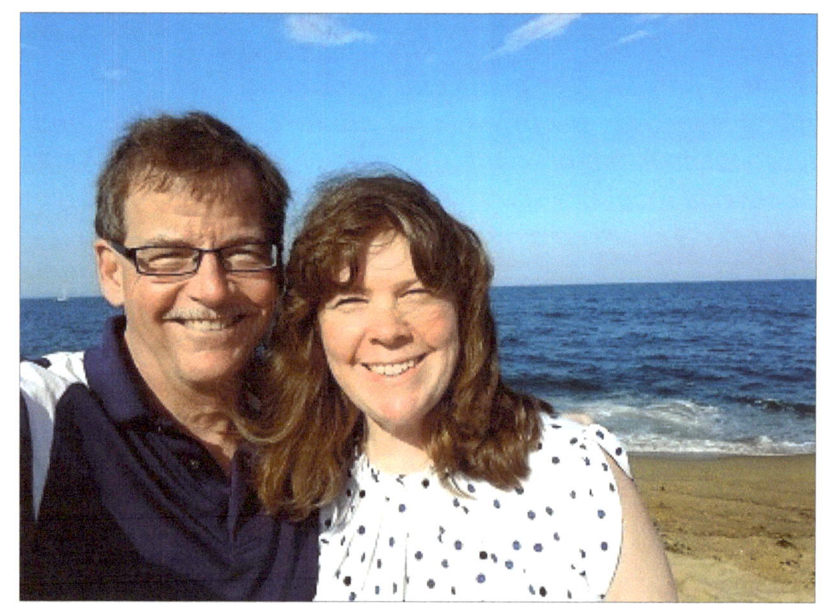

ABI, & stroke are welcome, as are family members, caregivers and anyone looking to learn more about brain injury." Though every injury is different, as is every outcome, we truly want all who are affected by brain injury in any way to find a safe haven at the TBI Hope Network.

If we could do it all over again, we would have started this as the Brain Injury Hope Network and been completely inclusive from the start. But we didn't know what we didn't know.

While Sarah and I help the gears to turn smoothly, The TBI Hope Network is just that – a worldwide network of members brought together by a common bond. If you've taken the time to read this far, you have been somehow connected to brain injury. If you have any thoughts about how we can better serve the brain injury community, we welcome you to share your thoughts. You have the power to help lift humanity higher.

~David & Sarah